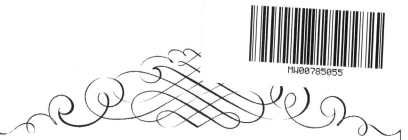
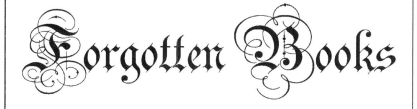

ISBN 978-1-332-91079-3
PIBN 10436774

# 1 MONTH OF
# FREE
# READING

## at

## www.ForgottenBooks.com

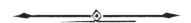

By purchasing this book you are eligible for one month membership to ForgottenBooks.com, giving you unlimited access to our entire collection of over 1,000,000 titles via our web site and mobile apps.

To claim your free month visit:

www.forgottenbooks.com/free436774

English
Français
Deutsche
Italiano
Español
Português

# www.forgottenbooks.com

**Mythology** Photography **Fiction**
Fishing Christianity **Art** Cooking
Essays Buddhism Freemasonry
Medicine **Biology** Music **Ancient
Egypt** Evolution Carpentry Physics
Dance Geology **Mathematics** Fitness
Shakespeare **Folklore** Yoga Marketing
**Confidence** Immortality Biographies
Poetry **Psychology** Witchcraft
Electronics Chemistry History **Law**
Accounting **Philosophy** Anthropology
Alchemy Drama Quantum Mechanics
Atheism Sexual Health **Ancient History**
**Entrepreneurship** Languages Sport
Paleontology Needlework Islam
**Metaphysics** Investment Archaeology
Parenting Statistics Criminology
**Motivational**

# RIFLE

### AND

# LIGHT INFANTRY TACTICS;

### FOR

### EXERCISE AND MANŒUVRES

#### OF

### Troops when acting as Light Infantry or Riflemen.

PREPARED UNDER THE DIRECTION OF THE WAR DEPARTMENT,

## BY BREVET-LIEUT.-COL. W. J. HARDEE, .C S. A.

### SCHOOLS OF THE SOLDIER AND COMPANY, INSTRUCTION FOR SKIRMISHERS,
### COMPLETE IN MATTER AND ILLUSTRATIONS.

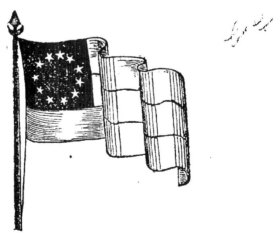

### NEW ORLEANS:
### H. P. LATHROP, PRINTER, 74 MAGAZINE ST.
### 1861.

- WAR DEPARTMENT;

March 29, 1855.

THE system of Tactics for Light Infantry and Riflemen, pre-pared under the direction of the War Department by Brevet Lieutenant Colonel William J. Hardee, of the Cavalry, having been approved by the President, is adopted for the instruction of he troops when acting as Light Infantry or Riflemen, and, under the Act of May 12, 1820, for the observance of the Militia when so employed.

JEFFERSON DAVIS,
*Secretary of War.*

# Rifle and Light Infantry Tactics.

## TITLE FIRST.

### ARTICLE FIRST.

*Formation of a Regiment in order of battle, or in line.*

1. A REGIMENT is composed of ten companies, which will habitually be posted from right to left, in the following order: first, sixth, fourth, ninth, third, eighth, fifth, tenth, seventh, second, according to the rank of the captains.

2. With a less number of companies the same principle will be observed, viz: the first captain will command the right company, the second captain the left company, the third captain the right centre company, and so on.

3. The companies thus posted will be designated from right to left, *first* company, *second* company, &c. This designation will be observed in the manœuvres.

4. The first two companies on the right, whatever their denomination, will form the *first division;* the next two companies the *second division;* and so on, to the left.

5. Each company will be divided into two equal parts, which will be designated as the first and second platoon, counting from the right; and each platoon, in like manner, will be subdivided into two sections.

6. In all exercises and manœuvres, every regiment, or part of a regiment, composed of two or more companies, will be designated as a battalion.

7. The color, with a guard to be hereinafter designated, will be posted on the left of the right centre battalion company. That company, and all on its right, will be denominated the *right wing* of the battalion; the remaining companies the *left wing*.

8. The formation of a regiment is in two ranks; and each company will be formed into two ranks, in the following manner: the corporals will be posted in the front rank, and on the right and left of platoons, according to the height; the tallest corporal and the tallest man will form the first file, the next two tallest men will form the second file, and so on to the last file, which will be composed of the shortest corporal and the shortest man.

9. The odd and even files, numbered as one, two, in the com-

pany, from right to left, will form groups of four men, who will be designated, *comrades in battle.*

10. The distance from one rank to another will be thirteen inches, measured from the breasts of the rear rank men to the backs or knapsacks of the front rank men.

11. For manœuvring, the companies of a battalion will always be equalized, by transferring men from the strongest to the weak. est companies.

### Posts of Company Officers, Sergeants and Corporals.

12. The company officers and sergeants are nine in number, and will be posted in the following manner:

13. The *captain* on the right of the company touching with the left elbow.

14. The *first sergeant* in the rear rank, touching with the left elbow, and covering the captain. In the manœuvres he will be denominated *covering sergeant,* or *right guide* of the company.

15. The remaining officers and sergeants will be posted as file closers, and two paces behind the rear rank.

16. The *first lieutenant,* opposite the centre of the fourth section.

17. The *second lieutenant,* opposite the centre of the first platoon.

18. The *third lieutenant,* opposite the centre of the second platoon.

19. The *second sergeant,* opposite the second file from the left of the company. In the manœuvres he will be designated *left guide* of the company.

20. The *third sergeant,* opposite the second file from the right of the second platoon.

21. The *fourth sergeant,* opposite the second file from the left of the first platoon.

22. The *fifth sergeant,* opposite the second file from the right of the first platoon.

23. In the left or tenth company of the battalion, the second sergeant will be posted in the front rank, and on the left of the battalion.

24. The corporals will be posted in the front rank, as prescribed No. 8.

25. Absent officers and sergeants will be replaced—officers by sergeants, and sergeants by corporals. The colonel may detach a first lieutenant from one company to command another, of which both the captain and first lieutenant are absent ; but this authority will give no right to a lieutenant to demand to be so detached.

### Posts of Field Officers and Regimental Staff.

26. The field officers, colonel, lieutenant colonel and major, are supposed to be mounted, and on active service shall be on horseback. The adjutant, when the battalion is manœuvering, will be on foot.

27. The colonel will take post thirty paces in rear of the file closers, and opposite the centre of the battalion. This distance will be reduced whenever there is a reduction in the front of the battalion.

28. The lieutenant colonel and the major will be opposite the centres of the right and left wings respectively, and twelve paces in rear of the file closers.

29. The adjutant and sergeant major will be opposite the right and left of the battalion, respectively, and eight paces in the rear of the file closets.

30. The adjutant and sergeant major will aid the lieutenant colonel and major, respectively, in the manœuvres.

31. The colonel, if absent, will be replaced by the lieutenant colonel, and the latter by the major. If all the field officers be absent, the senior captain will command the battalion ; but if either be present, he will not call the senior captain to act as field officer, except in case of evident necessity.

32. The quarter-master, surgeon, and other staff officers, in one rank, on the left of the colonel, and three paces in his rear.

33. The quarter-master sergeant, on a line with the front rank of the field music, and two paces on the right.

## Posts of Field Music and Band.

34. The buglers will be drawn up in four ranks, and posted twelve paces in rear of the file closers, the left opposite the centre of the left centry company. The senior principal musician will be two paces in front of the field music, and the other two paces in the rear.

35. The regimental band, if there be one, will be drawn up in two or four ranks, according to its numbers, and posted five paces in rear of the field music, having one of the principal musicians at its head.

## Color-guard.

35. In each battalion the color-guard will be composed of eight corporals, and posted on the left of the right centre company, of which company, for the time being, the guard will make a part.

36. The front rank will be composed of a sergeant, to be selected by the colonel, who will be called, for the time, *color-bearer*, with the two ranking corporals, respectively, on his right and left ; the rear rank will be composed of the three corporals next in rank ; and the three remaining corporals will be posted in their rear, and on the line of file closers. The left guide of the color-company, when these three last named corporals are in the rank of file closers, will be immediately on their left.

38. In battalions with less than five companies present, there will be no color-guard, and no display of colors, except it may be at reviews.

39. The corporals of the color-guard will be selected from those most distinguished for regularity and precision, as well in their positions under arms as in their marching. The latter advantage, and a just carriage of the person, are to be more particularly sought for in the selection of the color-bearer.

### General Guides.

40. There will be two *general* guides in each battalion, selected, for the time, by the colonel, from among the sergeants (other than first sergeants) the most distinguished for carriage under arms, and accuracy in marching.

41. These sergeants will be respectively denominated, in the manœuvres, *right general guide*, and *left general guide*, and be posted in the line of file closers ; the first in rear of the right, and the second in rear of the left flank of the battalion.

## INSTRUCTION OF THE BATTALION.

42. Every commanding officer is responsible for the instruction of his command. He will assemble the officers together for theoretical and practical instruction as often as he may judge necessary, and when unable to attend to this duty in person, it will be discharged by the officer next in rank.

43. Captains will be held responsible for the theoretical and practical instruction of their non-commissioned officers, and the adjutant for the instruction of the non-commissioned staff. To this end, they will require these tactics to be studied and recited lesson by lesson ; and when instruction is given on the ground, each non-commissioned officer, as he explains a movement, should be required to put it into practical operation.

44. The non-commissioned officers should also be practised in giving commands Each command, in a lesson, at the theoretical instruction, should first be given by the instructer, and then repeated, in succession, by the non-commissioned officers, so that while they become habituated to the commands, uniformity may be established in the manner of giving them.

45. In the school of the soldier, the company officers will be the instructors of the squads ; but if there be not a sufficient number of company officers present, intelligent sergeants may be substituted ; and two or three squads, under sergeant instructors, be superintended, at the same time, by an officer.

46. In the school of the company, the lieutenant colonel and the major, under the colonel, will be the principle instructors,

substituting frequently the captain of the company, and sometimes one of the lieutenants ; the substitute, as far as practicable, being superintented by one of the princincipals.

47. In the the school of the battalion, the brigadier general
may constitute himself the principal instructor, frequently substituting the colonel of the battalion, sometimes the lieutenant
colonel or major, and twice or thrice, in the same course of instruction, each of the three senior captains. In this school, also,
the substitute will always, if practicable, be superintended by the
brigadier general or the colonel, or (in case of a captain being
the instructor,) by the lieutenant colonel or major.

48. Individual instruction being the basis of the instruction
of companies, on which that of the regiment depends, and the
first principles having the greatest influence upon this individual instruction, classes of recruits should be watched with
the greatest care.

49. Instructors will explain, in a few clear and precise
words, the movements to be executed ; and not to overburden
the memory of the men, they will always use the same terms
to explain the same principles.

50. They should often join example to precept, should keep
up the attention of the men by an animated tone, and pass
rapidly from one movement to another, as soon as that which
they command has been executed in a satisfactory manner.

51. The sabre bayonet should only be fixed when required
to be used, either for attack or defence; the exercises and manœuvres will be executed without the bayonet.

52. In the movements which require the bayonet to be fixed,
the chief of the battalion will cause the signal *to fix bayonet*,
to be sounded ; at this signal the men will fix bayonets without command, and immediately replace their pieces in the
position they were before the signal.

## Instruction of Officers.

53. The instruction of officers can be perfected only by joining
theory to practice. The colonel will often practise them in
marching and in estimating distances, and he will carefully endeavor to cause them to take steps equal in length and swiftness.
They will also be exercised in the double quick step.

54. The instruction of officers will include all the Titles in this
system of drill, and such regulations as prescribe their duties in
peace and war.

55. Every officer will make himself perfectly acquainted with
the bugle signals.; and should, by practice, be enabled, if necessary, to sound them. This knowledge, so necessary in general
instruction, becomes of vital importance on actual service in the
field.

### Instruction of Sergeants.

56. As the discipline and efficiency of a company materially depend on the conduct and character of its sergeants, they should be selected with care, and properly instructed in all the duties appertaining to their rank.

57. Their theoretical instruction should include the School of the Soldier, the School of the Company, and the Drill for Skirmishers. They should likewise know all the details of service, and the regulations prescribing their duties in garrison and in campaign.

58. The captain selects from the corporals in his company those whom he judges fit to be admitted to the theoretical instruction of the sergeants.

### Instruction of Corporals.

59. Their theoretical instruction should include the School of the Soldier, and such regulations as prescribe their duties in garrison and in campaign.

60. The captain selects from his company a few privates, who may be admitted to the theoretical instruction of the corporals.

61. As the instruction of sergeants and corporals is intended principally to qualify them for the instruction of the privates, they should be taught not only to execute, but to explain intelligibly every thing they may be required to teach.

## COMMANDS.

There are three kinds.

62. The command of *caution*, which is *attention*.

63. The *preparatory command*, which indicates the movement which is to be executed.

64. The command of *execution*, such as *march* or *halt*, or, in the manual of arms, the part of command which causes an execution.

65. The tone of the command should be animated, distinct, and of a loudness proportioned to the number of men under instruction

66. The command *attention* is pronounced at the top of the voice, dwelling on the last syllable.

67. The command of *execution* will be pronounced in a tone firm and brief.

68. The commands of caution and the preparatory commands are herein distinguished by *italics*, those of execution by CAPITALS.

69. Those preparatory commands which, from their length, are difficult to be pronounced at once, must be divided into two or three parts, with an ascending progression in the tone of command, but always in such a manner that the tone of execution may be more energetic and elevated; the divisions are indicated by a hyphen. The parts of commands which are placed in a parenthesis, are not pronounced.

# TITLE SECOND.

---

# SCHOOL OF THE SOLDIER.

*General Rules and division of the School of the Soldier.*

1. The object of this school being the individual and progressive instruction of the recruits, the instructor never requires a movement to be executed until he has given an exact explanation of it; and he executes, himself, the movement which he commands, so as to join example to precept. He accustoms the recruit to take, by himself, the position which is explained—teaches him to rectify it only when required by his want of intelligence—and sees that all the movements are performed without precipitation.

2. Each movement should be understood before passing to another. After they have been properly executed in the order laid down in each lesson, the instructor no longer confines himself to that order; on the contrary, he should change it, that he may judge of the intelligence of the men.

3. The instructor allows the men to rest at the end of each part of the lessons, and oftener, if he thinks proper, especially at the commencement; for this purpose ho commands REST.

4. At the command Rest, the soldier is no longer required to preserve immobility, or to remain in his place. If the instructor wishes merely to relieve the attention of the recruit, he commands, *in place*—REST; the soldier is then not required to preserve his immobility, but he always keeps one of his feet in its place.

5. When the instructor wishes to commence the instruction, he commands—ATTENTION; at this command, the soldier takes his position, remains motionless, and fixes his attention

6. The *School of the Soldier* will be divided into three parts: the first, comprehending what ought to be taught to recruits without arms; the second, the manual of arms, the loading and firings; the third, the principles of alignment, the march by the front, the different steps, the march by the flank. the principles of wheeling, and those of change of direction; also, long marches in double quick time and the run

7. Each part will be divided into lessons, as follows:

### PART FIRST.

*Lesson* 1. Position of the soldier without arms: Eyes right, left and front.

*Lesson* 2. Facings.

*Lesson* 3. Principles of the direct step, in common and quick time.

*Lesson* 4. Principles of the direct step in double quick time, and the run.

### PART SECOND.

*Lesson* 1. Principles of shouldered arms.
*Lesson* 2. Manual of arms.
*Lesson* 3. To load in four times, and at will.
*Lesson* 4. Firings, direct, oblique, by file and by rank.
*Lesson* 5. To fire and load, kneeling and lying.
*Lesson* 6. Bayonet exercise.

### PART THIRD.

*Lesson* 1. Union of eight or twelve men for instruction in the principles of alignment.
*Lesson* 2. The direct march, the oblique march, and the different steps
*Lesson* 3. The march by the flank.
*Lesson* 4. Principles of wheeling and change of direction.
*Lesson* 5. Long marches in double quick time, and the run, with arms and knapsacks.

## PART FIRST.

8. This will be taught if practicable, to one recruit at a time; but three or four may be united when the number be great, compared with that of the instructors. In this case, the recruits will be placed in a single rank, at one pace from each other. In this part, the recruits will be without arms.

### LESSON I.

#### Position of the Soldier.

9. Heels on the same line, as near each other as the conformation of the man will permit ;
The feet turned out equally, and forming with each other something less than a right angle ;
The knees straight without stiffness ;
The body erect on the hips, inclining a little forward ;
The shoulders square and falling equally ;
The arms hanging naturally ;
The elbows near the body ;
The palm of the hand turned a little to the front, the little finger behind the seam of the pantaloons ;
The head erect and square to the front, without constraint ;
The chin near the stock, without covering it
The eyes fixed straight to the front, and striking the ground about the distance of fifteen paces.

REMARKS ON THE POSITION OF THE SOLDIER.

*Heels on the same line ;*

10. Because, if one were in rear of the other, the shoulder on that side would be thrown back, or the position of the soldier would be constrained.

*Heels more or less closed ;*

Because, men who are knock-kneed, or who have legs with large calves, cannot, without constraint, make their heels touch while standing.

*The feet equally turned out, and not forming too large an angle ;*

Because, if one foot were turned out more than the other, a shoulder would be deranged, and if both feet be too much turned out, it would not be practicable to incline the upper part of the body forward without rendering the whole position unsteady.

*Knees extended without stiffness ;*

Because, if stiffened, constraint and fatigue would be unavoidable.

*The body erect on the hips ;*

Because, it gives equilibrium to the position. The instructor will observe that many recruits have the bad habit of dropping a shoulder, of drawing in a side, or of advancing a hip, particularly the right, when under arms. These are defects he vill labor to correct.

*The upper part of the body inclining forward ;*

Because, commonly, recruits are disposed to do the reverse, to project the belly, and throw back the shoulders, when they wish to hold themselves erect, from which result great inconvenience in marching. The habit of inclining forward, the upper part of the body is so important to contract, that the instructor must enforce it at the beginning, particularly with recruits who have naturally the opposite habit.

*Shoulders square ;*

Because, if the shoulders be advanced beyond the line of the breast, and the back arched (the defect called *round-shouldered*, not uncommon among recruits,) the man cannot align himself, nor use his piece with address. It is important, then, to correct this defect, and necessary to that end that the coat should set easy about the shoulders and arm pits ; but in correcting this defect, the instructor will take care that the shoulders be not thrown too much to the rear, which would cause the belly to project, and the small of the back to be curved.

*The arms hanging naturally, elbows near the body, the palm of the
hand a little turned to the front, the little finger behind the seam
of the pantaloons ;*

Because, these positions are equally important to the *shoulder-
arms*, and to prevent the man from occupying more space in a
rank than is necessary to a free use of the piece ; they have,
moreover, the advantage of keeping in the shoulders.

*The face straight to the front, and without constraint ;*

Because, if there be stiffness in the latter position, it would
communicate itself to the whole of the upper part of the body,
embarrass its movements, and give pain and fatigue.

*Eyes direct to the front ;*

Because, this is the surest means of maintaining the shoulders
in line—an essential object, to be insisted on and attained.

11. The instructor having given the recruit the position of the
soldier without arms, will now teach him the turning of the head
and eyes. He will command :

1. *Eyes*—RIGHT. 2. FRONT.

12. At the word *right*, the recruit will turn the head gently,
so as to bring the inner corner of the left eye in a line with the
buttons of the coat, the eyes fixed on the line of the eyes of the
men in, or supposed to be in, the same rank.

13. At the second command, the head will resume the direct
or habitual position.

14. The movement of *Eyes*—LEFT will be executed by inverse
means.

15. The instructor will take particular care that the movement
of the head does not derange the squareness of the shoulders,
which will happen if the movement of the former be too sudden.

16. When the instructor shall wish the recruit to pass from the
state of attention to that of ease, he will command :

REST.

17. To cause a resumption of the habitual position, the instructor will command :

1. *Attention*. 2. SQUAD.

18. At the first word, the recruit will fix his attention ; at the
second, he will resume the prescribed position and steadiness.

LESSON II.
*Facings.*

19. Facing to the right and left will be executed in one *time*
or pause. The instructor will command :

1. *Squad*. 2. *Right* (or *left*)—FACE.

20. At the second command, raise the right foot slightly, turn

on the left heel, raising the toes a little, and then replace the right heel by the side of the left, and on the same line.

21. The full face to the rear (or front) will be executed in two *times*, or pauses. The instructor will command :

1. *Squad.* 2. ABOUT—FACE.

22. (*First time.*) At the word *about*, the recruit will turn on the left heel, bring the left toe to the front, carry the right foot to the rear, the hollow opposite to, and full three inches from, the left heel, the feet square to each other.

23. (*Second time.*) At the word *face*, the recruit will turn on both heels, raise the toes a little, extend the hams, face to the rear, bringing, at the same time, the right heel by the side of the left.

24. The instructor will take care that these motions do not derange the positon of the body.

LESSON III.

*Principles of the direct step.*

25. The length of the direct step, or pace, in common time, will be twenty-eight inches, reckoning from heel to heel, and in swiftness, at the rate of ninety in a minute.

26. The instructor, seeing the recruit confirmed in this position will explain to him the principle and mechanism of this step —placing himself six or seven paces from, and facing to the recruit. He will himself execute slowly the step in the way of illustration, and then command :

1. *Squad, forward.* 2. *Common time.* 3. MARCH.

27. At the first command, the recruit will throw the weight of the body on the right leg, without bending the left knee.

28. At the third command, he will smartly, but without a jerk, carry straight forward the left foot twenty-eight inches from the right, the sole near the ground, the ham extended, the toe a little depressed, and, as also the knee, slightly turned out; he will at the same time, throw the weight of the body forward, and plant flat the left foot, without shock, precisely at the distance where it finds itself from the right, when the weight of the body is brought forward, the whole of which will now rest on the advanced foot. The recruit will next, in like manner, advance the right foot and plant it as above, the heel twenty-eight inches from the heel of the left foot, and thus continue to march without crossing the legs, or striking the one against the other, without turning the shoulders, and preserving always the face direct to the front.

29. When the instructor shall wish to arrest the march, he will command ;

1. *Squad.* 2. HALT.

30. At the second command, which will be given at the in-

stant when either foot is coming to the ground, the foot in the rear will be brought up, and planted by the side of the other without shock·

31. The instructor will indicate, from time to time, to the re. cruit, the cadence of the step by giving the command *one* at the. instant of raising the foot, and *two* at the instant it ought to be planted, observing the cadence of ninety steps in a minute.    This method will contribute greatly to impress upon the mind the two motions into which the step is naturally divided.

32. Common time will be employed only in the first and second parts of the School of the Soldier.    As soon as the recruit has acquired steadiness, has become established in the principles of shouldered arms, and in the mechanism, length and swiftness of the step in common time, he will be practised only in quick time, the double quick time, and the run.

33. The principles of the step in quick time are the same as for common time, but its swiftness is at the rate of one hundred and ten steps per minute.

34. The instructor wishing the squad to march in quick time, will command:

1. *Squad, forward.*  2. MARCH.

LESSON IV.

*Principles of the Double Quick Step.*

35. The length of the double quick step is thirty-three inches, and its swiftness at the rate of one hundred and sixty-five steps per minute.

36. The instructor wishing to teach the recruits the principles and mechanism of the double quick step, will command:

1. *Double Quick Step.*  2. MARCH.

37. At the first command the recruit will raise his hands to a level with his hips, the hands closed, the nails towards the body, the elbows to the rear.

38. At the second command, he will raise to the front his left leg bent, in order to give to the knee the greatest elevation, the part of the leg between the knee and the instep vertical, the toe depressed; he will then replace his foot in its former position; with the right leg he will execute what has just been prescribed for the left, and the alternate movement of the legs will be con· tinued until the command:

1. *Squad.*  2. HALT.

39. At the second command, the recruit will bring the foot which is raised by the side of the other, and dropping at tbo same time his hands by his side, will resume the position of the soldier without arms.

40. The instructor placing himself seven or eight paces from,

and facing the recruit, will indicate the cadence by the commands, **one** and *two*, given alternately at the instant each foot should be brought to the ground, which at first will be in common time, but its rapidity will be gradually augmented.

41. The recruit being sufficiently established in the principles of this step, the instructer will command :

1. *Squad, forward.* 2. *Double quick.* 3 MARCH.

42. At the first command, the recruit will throw the weight o, his body on the right leg.

43. At the second command he will place his arms as indicated No. 37

44. At the third command, he will carry forward the left foot, the leg slightly bent, the knee somewhat raised—will plant his left foot, the toe first, thirty-three inches from the right, and with the right foot will then execute what has just been prescribed for the left. This alternate movement of the legs will take place by throwing the weight of the body on the foot that is planted, and by allowing a natural. oscillatory motion to the arms.

45. The double quick step may be executed with different degrees of swiftness. Under urgent circumstances the cadence of the step may be increased to one hundred and eighty per minute. At this rate a distance of four thousand yards would be passed over in about twenty-five minutes.

46. The recruits will be exercised also in running.

47. The principles are the same as for the double quick step, the only difference consisting in a greater degree of swiftness.

48. It is recommended in marching at double quick time, or the run, that the men should breathe as much as possible through the nose, keeping the mouth closed. Experience has proved that, by conforming to this principle, a man can pass over a much longer distance, and with less fatigue.

## PART SECOND.

### GENERAL RULES.

49. The instructor will not pass the men to this second part until they shall be well established in the position of the body, and in the manner of marching at the different steps.

50. He will then unite four men, whom he will place in the same rank, elbow to elbow, and instruct them in the position of shouldered arms, as follows:

### LESSON I.

#### *Principles of Shouldered Arms.*

51. The recruit being placed as explained in the first lesson of the first part, the instructor will cause him to bend the right arm slightly, and place the piece in it, in the following manner:

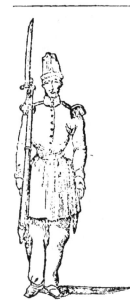

52. The piece in the right hand—the barrel nearly vertical and resting in the hollow
of the shoulder—the guard to the front, the
arm hanging nearly at its full length near
the body ; the thumb and fore finger embracing the guard, the remaining fingers
closed together, and grasping the swell of
the stock just under the cock, which rests
on the little finger.

53. Recruits are frequently seen with
natural defects in the conformation of the
shoulders, breast and hips. These the instructor will labor to correct in the lessons
without arms, and afterwards, by steady
endeavors, so that the appearance of the
pieces, in the same line, may be uniform,
and this without constraint to the men in
their positions.

54. The instructor will have occasion to
remark that recruits, on first bearing arms, are liable to derange
their positions by lowering the right shoulder and the right hand,
or by sinking the hip and spreading out the elbows.

55. He will be careful to correct all these faults by continually
rectifying the position ; he will sometimes take away the piece
to replace it the better ; he will avoid fatiguing the recruits too
much in the beginning, but labor by degrees to render this position so natural and easy that they may remain in it a long time
without fatigue.

56. Finally, the instructor will take great care that the piece,
at a shoulder, be not carried too high nor too low ; if too high,
the right elbow would spread out, the soldier would occupy too
much space in his rank, and the piece be made to waver ; if too
low the files would be too much closed, the soldier would not
have the necessary space to handle his piece with facility, the
right arm would become too much fatigued, and draw down the
shoulder.

57. The instructor, before passing to the second lesson, will
cause to be repeated the movements of *eyes right, left*, and *front*,
and the *facings*.

### LESSON II.

#### Manual of Arms.

58. The manual of arms will be taught to four men, placed at
first, in one rank, elbow to elbow, and afterwards in two ranks.

59. Each command will be executed in one *time* (or pause,)
but this time will be divided into motions, the better to make
known the mechanism.

60. the rate (or swiftness) of each motion, in the manual of

arms, with the exceptions herein indicated, is fixed at the ninetieth part of a minute; but in order not to fatigue the attention, the instructor will, at first, look more particularly to the execution of the motions, without re-quiring a nice observance of the cadence, to which he will bring the re-cruits progressively, and after they shall have become a little familiarized with the handling of the piece.

61. As the motions relative to the cartridge, to the rammer, and to the fixing and unfixing of the bayonet, cannot be executed at the rate prescribed, nor even with a uniform swiftness, they will not be subjected to that cadence. The instructor will, however, labor to cause these motions to be executed with promptness, and, above all, with regularity.

62. The last syllable of the command will decide the brisk execution of the first motion of each time (or pause) The commands *two, three* and *four*, will decide the brisk execution of the other motions. As soon as the recruits shall well comprehend the positions of the several motions of a time, they will be taught to execute the time without resting on its different motions; the mechanism of the time will nevertheless be observed, as well as to give a perfect use of the piece, as to avoid the sinking of, or slurring over, either of the motions.

63. The manual of arms will be taught in the following pro-gression: The instructor will command:

*Support*—Arms. (*One time and three motions.*)

**64.** (*First motion*) Bring the piece, with the right hand, perpendicularly to the front and between the eyes, the barrel to the rear; seize the piece with the left hand at the lower band, raise this hand as high as the chin, and seize the piece at the same time with the right hand four inches below the cock.

65 (*Second motion.*) Turn the piece with the right hand, the barrel to the front; carry the piece to the left shoulder, and pass the fore-arm extended on the breast between the right hand and the cock; support the cock against the left fore-arm, the left hand resting on the right breast.

66. (*Third motion.*) Drop the right hand by the side.

67. When the instructor may wish to give repose in this position, he will command:

REST.

68. At this command, the recruits will bring up smartly the right hand to the handle of the piece (small of the stock,) when they will not be required to pre-serve silence, or steadiness of position.

69. When the instructor may wish the recruits to pass from this position to that of silence and steadiness, he will command:

1. *Attention.* 2. SQUAD.

70. At the second word, the recruits will resume the position of the third motion of *support arms.*

2

*Shoulder—*Arms.

*One time and three motions.*

71. (*First motion.*) Grasp the piece with the right hand under and against the left fore-arm ; seize it with the left hand at the lower band, the thumb extended ; detach the piece slightly from the shoulder, the left fore-arm along the stock.

72. (*Second motion.*) Carry the piece vertically to the right shoulder with both hands, the rammer to the front, change the position of the right hand so as to embrace the guard with the thumb and fore finger, slip the left hand to the height of the shoulder, the fingers ex. tended and joined, the right arm nearly straight.

73. (*Third motion.*) Drop the left hand quickly by the side.

*Present—*Arms.

*One time and two motions.*

74. (*First motion.*) With the right hand bring the piece erect before the centre of the body, the rammer to the front; at the same time seize the piece with the left hand half-way between the guide sight and lower band, the thumb extended along the barrel and against the stock, the fore-arm horizontal and resting against the body, the hand as high as the elbow.

75. (*Second motion.*) Grasp the small of the stock with the right hand below and against the guard.

*Shoulder—*Arms.   (*One time and two motions.*)

76. (*First motion.*) Bring the piece to the right shoulder, at the same time change the position of the right hand so as to embrace the guard with the thumb and forefinger, slip up the left hand to the height of the shoulder, the fingers extended and joined, the right arm nearly straight.

77. (*Second motion.*) Drop the left hand quickly by the side.

*Order—*Arms.   (*One time and two motions.*)

78. (*First motion.*)  Seize the piece briskly with the left hand near the upper band, and detach it slightly from the shoulder with the right hand ; loosen the grasp of the right hand, lower the piece with the left, reseize the piece with the right hand above the lower band, the little finger in rear of the barrel, the butt about four inches from the ground, the right hand supported against the hip, drop the left hand by the side.

79. (*Second motion.*) Let the piece slip through the right hand to the ground by opening slightly the fingers, and take the position about to be described.

### Position of Order Arms.

80. The hand low, the barrel between the thumb and fore-finger extended along the stock; the other fingers extended and joined; the muzzle about two inches from the right shoulder; the rammer in front; the toe (or beak) of the butt, against, and in a line with, the toe of the right foot, the barrel perpendicular.

81. When the instructor may wish to give repose in this position, he will command:

### REST.

82. At this command, the recruits will not be required to preserve silence or steadiness.

83. When the instructor may wish the recruits to pass from this position to that of silence and steadiness, he will command:

### 1. *Attention.* 2. SQUAD.

84. At the second word, the recruits will resume the position or *order arms*.

### *Shoulder—*ARMS. (*One time and two motions.*)

85. (*First motion.*) Raise the piece vertically with the right hand to the height of the right breast, and opposite the shoulder, the elbow close to the body; seize the piece with the left hand below the right, and drop quickly the right hand to grasp the piece at the swell of the stock, the thumb and fore finger embracing the guard; press the piece against the shoulder with the left hand, the right arm nearly straight.

86. (*Second motion.*) Drop the left hand quickly by the side.

### Load in nine times.

### 1. LOAD.* (*One time and one motion.*)

87. Grasp the piece with the left hand as high as the right elbow, and bring it vertically opposite the middle of the body, shift the right hand to the upper band, place the butt between the feet, the barrel to the front; seize it with the left hand near the muzzle, which should be three inches from the body; carry the right hand to the cartridge box.

### 2. *Handle—*CARTRIDGE. (*One time, one motion.*)

88. Seize the cartridge with the thumb and next two fingers, and place it between the teeth.

### 3. *Tear—*CARTRIDGE. (*One time and one motion.*)

89. Tear the paper to the powder, hold the cart-

---

*Whenever the loadings and firings are to be executed, the instructor will cause the cartridge boxes to be brought to the front.

ridge upright between the thumb and first two fingers near the top; in this position place it in front of and near the muzzle—the back of the hand to the front.

### 4. Charge—CARTRIDGE.

*One time and one motion.*

90. Empty the powder into the barrel; disengage the ball from the paper with the right hand and the thumb and first two fingers of the left; insert it into the bore, the pointed end uppermost, and press it down with the right thumb; seize the head of the rammer with the thumb and fore finger of the right hand, the other fingers closed, the elbows near the body.

### 5. Draw—RAMMER.

*One time and three motions.*

91. (*First motion.*) Half draw the rammer by extending the right arm; steady it in this position with the left thumb; grasp the rammer near the muzzle with the right hand, the little finger uppermost, the nails to the front, the thumb extended along the rammer.

92. (*Second motion.*) Clear the rammer from the pipes by again extending the arm; the rammer in the prolongation of the pipes.

93. (*Third motion*) Turn the rammer, the little end of the rammer passing near the left shoulder: place the head of the rammer on the ball, the back of the hand to the front.

### 6. Ram—CARTRIDGE.

*One time and one motion.*

94. Insert the rammer as far as the right, and steady it in this position with the thumb of the left hand; seize the rammer at the small end with the thumb and fore-finger of the right hand, the back of the hand to the front; press the ball home, the elbows near the body.

### 7. Return—RAMMER.

*One time and three motions.*

95. (*First motion.*) Draw the rammer half-way out, and steady it in this position with the left thumb; grasp it near the muzzle with the right hand, the little finger uppermost, the nails to the front, the thumb along the rammer; clear the rammer from the bore by extending the arm, the nails to the front, the rammer in the prolongation of the bore.

96. (*Second motion.*) Turn the rammer, the head of the rammer passing near the left shoulder, and insert it in the pipes until the right hand reaches the muzzle, the nails to the front.

97. (*Third motion.*) Force the rammer home by placing the little finger of the right hand on the head of the rammer; pass the left hand down the barrel to the extent of the arm, without depressing the shoulder.

## 8. Prime.*

*One time and two motions.*

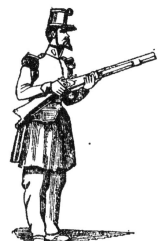

93. (*First motion.*) With the left hand raise the piece till the hand is as high as the eye, grasp the small of the stock with the right hand; half face to the right; p'ace, at the same time, the right foot behind and at right angles with the left; the hollow of the right foot against the left heel. Slip the left hand down to the lower band, the thumb along the stock, the left elbow against the body, bring the piece to the right side, the butt below the right fore-arm—the small of the stock against the body and two inches below the right breast, the barrel upwards, the muzzle on a level with the eye.

99. (*Second motion.*) Half cock with the thumb of the right hand, the fingers supported against the guard and the small of the stock—remove the old cap with one of the fingers of the right hand, and with the thumb and fore finger of the same hand take a cap from the pouch, place it on the nipple, and press it down with the thumb; seize the small of the stock with the right hand.

## 9. Shoulder—Arms.

*One time and two motions.*

100. (*First motion.*) Bring the piece to the right shoulder and support it there with the left hand, face to the front; bring the right heel to the side of and on a line with the left; grasp the piece with the right hand as indicated in the position of *shoulder arms.*

101. (*Second motion.*) Drop the left hand quickly by the side.

### Ready.

*One time and three motions.*

102. (*First motion.*) Raise the piece slightly with the right hand, making a half face to the right on the left heel; carry the right foot to the rear, and place it at right angles to the left, the hollow of it opposite to, and against the left heel; grasp the piece with the left hand at the lower band and detach it slightly from the shoulder.

---

*If Maynard's primer be used, the command will be, *load in eight times,* and the eighth command will be, *shoulder arms,* and executed from *return rammer,* in one and two motions as follows :

(*First motion.*) Raise the piece with the left hand, and take the position of shoulder arms as indicated No. 76.

(*Second motion*) Drop the left hand quickly by the side.

103. (*Second motion.*) Bring down the piece with both hands, the barrel upwards, the left thumb extended along the stock, the butt below the right fore-arm, the small of the stock against the body and two inches below the right breast, the muzzle as high as the eye, the left elbow against the side; place at the same time the right thumb on the head of the cock, the other fingers under and against the guard.

104. (*Third motion.*) Cock, and seize the piece at the small of the stock without deranging the position of the butt.

AIM. (Front rank.)
*One time and one motion.*

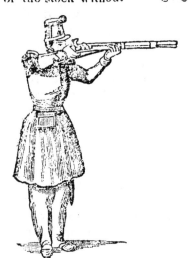

105. Raise the piece with both hands, and support the butt against the right shoulder; the left elbow down the right as high as the shoulder; incline the head upon the butt, so that the right eye may perceive quickly the notch of the hausse, the front sight, and the object aimed at; the left eye closed, the right thumb extended along the stock, the fore finger on the trigger.

106. When recruits are formed in two ranks to execute the firings, the front rank men will raise a little less the right elbow, in order to facilitate the aim of the rear rank men.

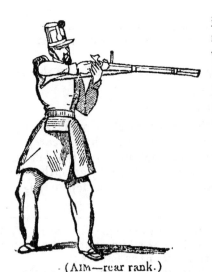

(Aim—rear rank.)

107 The rear rank men, in aiming, will each carry the right foot about eight inches to the right, and towards the left heel of the man next on the right, inclining the upper part of the body forward.

FIRE. (*One time, one motion.*)

108. Press the fore finger against the trigger, fire, without lowering or turning the head, and remain in this position.

109. Instructors will be careful to observe when the men fire that they aim at some distinct object, and that the barrel be so directed that the line of fire and the line of sight being the same vertical plane. They will often cause the firing to be

executed on ground of different inclinations, in order to accustom the men to fire at objects either above or below them.

## LOAD.

*One time and one motion.*

110. Bring down the piece with both hands, at the same time face to the front and take the position of *load* as indicated No. 87. Each rear rank man will bring his right foot by the side of the left.

111. The men being in this position, the instructor will cause the loading to be continued by the commands and means prescribed No. 87. and following.

112. If, after firing, the instructor should not wish the recruits to reload, he will command:

### Shoulder—ARMS.

*One time and one motion.*

113. Throw up the piece briskly with the left hand and resume the position of *shoulder arms*, at the same time face to the front, turning on the left heel, and bring the right heel on a line with the left.

114. To accustom the recruits to wait for the command *fire*, the instructor, when they are in the position of *aim*, will command:

### Recover—ARMS.

*One time and one motion.*

115. At the first part of the command, withdraw the finger from the trigger; at the command *arms*, retake the position of the third motion of *ready*.

116. The recruits being in the position of the third motion of *ready*, if the instructor should wish to bring them to a shoulder, he will command:

### SHOULDER—ARMS.

*One time and one motion.*

117. At the command *shoulder*, place the thumb upon the cock, the fore-finger on the trigger, half-cock. and seize the small of the stock with the right hand. At the command *arms*, bring up the piece briskly to the right shoulder, and retake the position of shoulder arms.

118. The recruits being at shoulder arms, when the instructor shall wish to fix bayonets, he will command:

### Fix—BAYONET.

*One time and three motions.*

119. (*First motion.*) Grasp the piece with the left hand at the height of the shoulder, and detach it slightly from the shoulder with the right hand.

120. (*Second motion.*) Quit the piece with the right hand, lower it with the left hand, opposite the middle of the body, and place the butt between the feet without shock; the rammer to the rear, the barrel vertical, the muzzle three inches from the body; seize it with the right hand at the upper band, and carry the left hand reversed to the handle of the sabre-bayonet.

121. (*Third motion.*) Draw the sabre-bayonet from the scabbard and fix it on the extremity of the barrel; seize the piece with the left hand, the arm extended, the right hand at the upper band.

### Shoulder—ARMS.

*One time and two motions.*

122. (*First motion.*) Raise the piece with the left hand and place it against the right shoulder, the rammer to the front; seize the piece at the same time with the right hand at the swell of the stock, the thumb and fore finger embracing the guard, the right arm nearly extended.

123. (*Second motion.*) Drop briskly the left hand by the side.

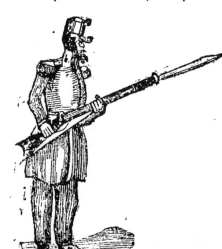

### Charge—BAYONET.

*One time and two motions.*

124. (*First motion.*) Raise the piece slightly with the right hand and make a half face to the right on the left heel; place the hollow of the right foot opposite to, and three inches from the left heel, the feet square: seize the piece at the same time with the left hand a little above the lower band.

125. (*Second motion*)— Bring down the piece with both hands, the barrel uppermost, the left elbow against the body; seize the small of the stock, at the same time, with the right hand, which will be supported against the hip; the point of the sabre-bayonet as high as the eye.

### Shoulder—ARMS.

*One time and two motions.*

126. (*First motion.*) Throw up the piece briskly with the left hand in facing to the front, place it against the right shoulder, the rammer to the front; turn the right hand so as to embrace the guard, slide the left hand to the height of the shoulder, the right hand nearly extended.

127. (*Second motion.*) Drop the left hand smartly by the side.

## Trail—Arms.

*One time and two motions.*

128. (*First motion.*) The same as the first motion of *order arms.*

129. (*Second motion*) Incline the muzzle slightly to the front, the butt to the rear and about four inches from the ground. The right hand supported at the hip, will so hold the piece th t the rear rank men may not touch with their bayonets the men in the front rank.

## Shoulder—Arms.

130. At the command *shoulder*, raise the piece perpendicularly in the right hand, the little finger in the rear of the barrel; at the command *arms*, execute what has been prescribed for the *shoulder* from the position of *order arms.*

## Unfix—Bayonet.

*One time and three motions.*

131. (*First and second motions.*) The same as the first and second motions of *fix bayonet*, except that, at the end of the second command, the thumb of the right hand will be placed on the spring of the sabre-bayonet, and the left hand will embrace the handle of the sabre-bayonet and the barrel, the thumb extended 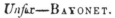 along the blade.

132 (*Third motion.*) Press the thumb of the right hand on the spring, wrest off the sabre-bayonet, turn it to the right, the edge to the front, lower the guard until it touches the right hand, which will seize the back and the edge of the blade between the thumb and first two fingers, the other fingers holding the piece ; change the position of the hand without quitting the handle, return the sabre bayonet to the scabbard, and seize the piece with the left hand, the arm extended.

## Shoulder—Arms.

*One time and two motions.*

133. (*First motion.*) The same as the first motion from *fix bayonet.* No. 122.

134. (*Second motion*) The same as the second motion from *fix, bayonet.* No. 123.

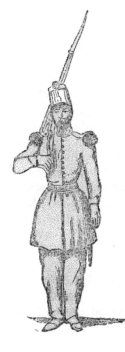

Secure—ARMS.

*One time and three motions.*

135. (*First motion.*) The same as the first motion of *support arms*, No. 64 except with the right hand seize the piece at the small of the stock.

136. (*Second motion*) Turn the piece with both hands, the barrel to the front; bring it opposite the left shoulder, the butt against the hip, the left hand at the lower band, the thumb as high as the chin and extended on the rammer; the piece erect and detached from the shoulder, the left fore arm against the piece.

137. (*Third motion*) Reverse the piece, pass it under the half arm, the left hand remaining at the lower band. the thumb on the rammer to prevent it from sliding out, the little finger resting against the hip, the right hand falling at the same time by the side.

Shoulder—ARMS.

*One time and three motions.*

138. (*First motion.*) Raise the piece with the left hand, and seize it with the right hand at the small of the stock. The piece erect and detached from the shoulder, the butt against the hip, the left fore arm along the piece.

139. (*Second motion*) The same as the second motion of *shoulder arms from a support.*

140. (*Third motion.*) The same as the third motion of *shoulder arms from a support.*

Right shoulder shift—ARMS.

*One time and two motions.*

141. (*First motion.*) Detach the piece perpendicularly from the shoulder with the right hand, and seize it with the left between the lower band and guide-sight, raise the piece, the left hand at the height of the shoulder and four inches from it; place, at the same time, the right hand on the butt, the beak between the first two fingers, the other two fingers under the butt plate.

142. (*Second motion*) Quit the piece with the left hand, raise and place the piece on the right shoulder with the right hand,

'the lock plate upwards; let fall, at the same time, the left hand by the side.

## Shoulder — ARMS.

*One time and two motions.*

143. (*First motion.*) Raise the piece perpendicularly by extending the right arm to its full length, the rammer to the front, at the same time seize the piece with the left hand between the lower band and guide sight.

144. (*Second motion.*) Quit the butt with the right hand, which will immediately embrace the guard, lower the piece to the position of shoulder arms, slide up the left hand to the height of the shoulder, the fingers extended and closed. Drop the left hand by the side.

145. The men being at support arms, the instructor will sometimes cause pieces to be brought to the right shoulder. To this effect, he will command:

## Right shoulder shift—ARMS.

*One time and two motions.*

146. (*First motion.*) Seize the piece with the right hand, below and near the left fore-arm, place the left hand under the butt, the heel of the butt between the first two fingers.

147. (*Second motion.*) Turn the piece with the left hand, the lock plate upwards, carry it to the right shoulder, the left hand still holding the butt, the muzzle elevated: hold the piece in this position and place the right hand upon the butt as is prescribed No. 141, and let fall the left hand by the side.

## Support—ARMS.

*One time and two motions.*

148. (*First motion.*) The same as the first motion of *shoulder arms*, No. 143.

149. (*Second motion.*) Turn the piece with both hands, the barrel to the front, carry it opposite the left shoulder, slip the right hand to the small of the stock, place the left fore-arm extended on the breast as is prescribed No. 65, and let fall the right hand by the side.

## Arms—AT WILL.

*One time and one motion.*

150. At this command, carry the piece at pleasure on either shoulder, with one or both hands, the muzzle elevated.

## Shoulder—ARMS.

*One time and one motion.*

151. At this command, retake quickly the position of shoulder arms.

152. The recruits being at ordered arms, when the instructor

shall wish to cause the pieces to be placed on the ground, he will command :

### Ground—ARMS.

*One time and two motions.*

153. (*First motion*) Turn the piece with the right hand, the barrel to the left, at the same time seize the cartridge box with the left hand, bend the body, advance the left foot, the heel opposite the lower ba. d ; lay the piece on the ground with the right hand, the toe of the butt on a line with the right toe, the knees slightly bent, the right heel raised.

154. (*Second motion*) Rise up, bring the left foot by the side of the right, quit the cartridge box with the left hand, and drop the hands hy. the side.

### Raise—ARMS.

*One time and two motions.*

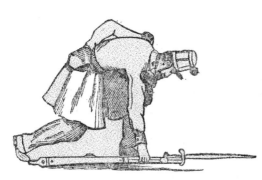

155. (*First motion.*) Seize the cartridge box with the left hand, bend the body, advance the left foot opposite the lower band, and seize the piece with the right hand.

156. (*Second motion.*) Raise the piece, bringing the left foot by the side of the right ; turn the piece with the right hand, the rammer to the front ; at the same time quit the cartridge box with the left hand, and drop this hand by the side.

### Inspection of Arms.

157. The recruits being at *ordered arms*, and having the sabre bayonet in the scabbard, if the instructor wishes to cause an inspection of arms, he will command :

### Inspection—ARMS.

*One time and two motions.*

158. (*First motion.*) Seize the piece with the left hand below and near the upper band, carry it with both hands opposite the middle of the body, the butt between the feet, the rammer to the rear, the barrel vertical, the muzzle about three inches from the body ; carry the left hand reversed to the sabre-bayonet, draw it from the scabbard and fix it on the barrel ; grasp the piece with the left hand below and near the upper band, seize the rammer with the thumb and fore-finger of the right hand bent, the other fingers closed.

159. (*Second motion.*) Draw the rammer as has been ex-

plained in *loading*, and let it glide to the bottom of the bore, re-place the piece with the left hand opposite the right shoulder, and retake the position of *ordered arms*.

160. The instructor will then inspect in succession the piece of each recruit, in passing along the front of the rank. Each, as the instructor reaches him, will raise smartly his piece with his right hand, seize it with the left between the lower band and guide sight, the lock to the front, the left hand at the height of the chin, the piece opposite to the left eye ; the instructor will take it with the right hand at the handle, and, after inspecting it, will return it to the recruit, who will receive it back with the right hand, and replace it in the position of *ordered arms*.

161. When the instructor shall have passed him, each recruit will retake the position prescribed at the command *inspection arms*, return the rammer, and resume the position of *ordered arms*.

162. If, instead of *inspection of arms*, the instructor should merely wish to cause bayonets to be fixed, he will command :

Fix—BAYONET.

163. Take the position indicated, No. 158, fix bayonets as has been explained, and immediately resume the position of *ordered arms*.

164. If it be the wish of the instructor, after firing, to ascertain whether the pieces have been discharged, he will command:

Spring—RAMMERS.

165. Put the rammer in the barrel as has been explained above, and immediately retake the position of *ordered arms*.

166. The instructor, for the purpose stated, can take the rammer by the small end, and spring it in the barrel, or cause each recruit to make it ring in the barrel.

167. Each recruit, after the instructor passes him, will return rammer, and resume the position of *ordered arms*.

## REMARKS ON THE MANUAL OF ARMS.

168. The manual of arms frequently distorts the persons of recruits before they acquire ease and confidence in the several positions. The instructor will therefore frequently recur to elementary principles in the course of the lessons.

169. Recruits are also extremely liable to curve the sides and back, and to derange the shoulders, especially in loading. Consequently, the instructor will not cause them to dwell too long, at a time, in one position.

170. When, after some days of exercise in the manual of arms, the four men shall be well established in their use, the instructor will always terminate the lesson by marching the men for some time in one rank, and at one pace apart, in common and quick time, in order to confirm them more and more in the mechanism

of the step ; he will also teach them to mark time and to change step, which will be executed in the following manner :

### To mark time.

171. The four men marching in the direct step, the instructor will command :

1. *Mark time.*  2. MARCH.

172. At the second command, which will be given at the instant a foot is coming to the ground, the recruits will make a semblance of marching, by bringing the heels by the side of each other, and observing the cadence of the step, by raising each foot alternately without advancing.

173. The instructor wishing the direct step to be resumed, will command :

1. *Forward.*  2. MARCH.

174. At the second command, which will be given as prescribed above, the recruits will retake the step of twenty-eight inches

### To change step.

175. The squad being in march, the instructor will command:

1. *Change step.*  2. MARCH.

176. At the second command, which will be given at the instant either foot is coming to the ground, bring the foot which is in rear by the side of that which is in front, and step off again with the foot which was in front.

### To march backwards.

177. The instructor wishing the squad to march backwards, will command :

1. *Squad backward.*  2. MARCH.

178. At the second command, the recruits will step off smartly with the left foot fourteen inches to the rear, reckoning from heel to heel, and so on with the feet in succession till the command *halt,* which will always be preceded by the caution *squad.* The men will halt at this command, and bring back the foot in front by the side of the other.

179. This step will always be executed in quick time.

180. The instructor will be watchful that the recruits march straight to the rear, and that the erect position of the body and the piece be not deranged.

### LESSON III.

#### To load in four times.

181. The object of this lesson is to prepare the recruits to load at will, and to cause them to distinguish the times which require the greatest regularity and attention, such as *charge catridge, ram catridge,* and *prime.* It will be divided as follows :

182. The first time will be executed at the end of the command ; the three others at the commands, *two*, *three*, and *four*.
The instructor will command :

> 1. *Load in four times.*  2. LOAD.

183. Execute the times to include charge catridge.

> TWO.

. 184. Execute the time to include ram oatridge.

> THREE.

185. Execute the times to include prime..

> FOUR.

186. Execute the time of *shoulder arms*..

> *To load at will.*

187. The iustructor will next teach loading at will, which will be execu ed as loading in four times, but continued, and without reating on either of the times.  He will command :

> 1. *Load at will..*  2. LOAD.

188. The instructor will habituate the recruits, by degrees, to load with the greatest possible promptitude, each without regulating himself by his neighbor, and above all, without waiting for him.

189. The cadence prescribed No· 60, is not applicable to loading in four times or at will.

## LESSON IV.

### *Firings.*

190. The firings are direct or oblique, and will be executed as follows :

> #### *The direct fire.*

191. The instructor will give the following commands :

> 1. *Fire by squad.* 2. *Squad.* 3. READY. 4. AIM. 5. FIRE. 6. LOAD.

192. These several commands will be executed as has been prescribed in the *Manual of Arms*.  At the third command, the men will come to the position of *ready* as heretofore explained. At the fourth they will aim according to the rank in which each may find himself placed, the rear rank men inclining forward a little the upper part of the body, in order that their pieces may reach as much beyond the front rank as possible.

193. At the sixth command, they will load their pieces and return immediately to the position of *ready*.

194. The instructor will recommence the firing by the command :

> 1. *Squad.* 2. AIM. 3. FIRE. 4. LOAD.

195. When the instructor wishes the firing to cease, he will command :

*Cease firing.*

196. At this command, the men will cease firing, but will load their pieces if unloaded, and afterwards bring them to a shoulder.

*Oblique firings.*

197. The oblique firings will be executed to the right and left, and by the same commands as the direct fire, with this single difference—the command *aim* will always be preceded by the caution, *right* or *left oblique.*

*Position of the two ranks in the oblige fire to the right.*

198. At the command *ready,* the two ranks will execute what has been prescribed for the direct line.

199 At the cautionary command, *right oblique,* the two ranks will throw back the right shoulder and look steadily at the object to be hit.

200. At the command *aim,* each front rank man will aim to the right without deranging the feet ; each rear rank man will advance the left foot about eight inches towards the right heel of the man next on the right of his file leader, and aim to the right, inclining the upper part of the body forward and bending a little the left knee.

*Position of the two ranks in the oblique fire to the left.*

201. At the cautionary command *left oblique,* the two ranks will throw back the left shoulder and look steadily at the object to be hit.

202. At the command *aim,* the front rank will take aim to the left without deranging the feet ; each man in the rear rank will advance the right foot about eight inches towards the right heel of the man next on the right of his file leader, and aim to the left, inclining the upper part of the body forward and bending a little the right knee.

203. In both cases, at the command *load,* the men of each rank will come to the position of load as prescribed in the direct fire ; the rear rank then bringing back the foot which is to the right and front by the side of the other. Each man will continue to load as if isolated.

*To fire by file.*

204. The fire by file will be executed by the two ranks, the files of which will fire successively, and without regulating on each other, except for the first fire.

205. The instructor will command :

1. *Fire by file.* 2. *Squad.* 3. READY 4. COMMENCE FIRING.

206. At the third command, the two two ranks will take the position prescribed in the direct fire.

207. At the fourth command, the file on the right will aim and fire ; the rear rank man in aiming will take the position indica- ted No. 107.

'208· The men of this file will load their pieces briskly and fire a second time; re-load and fire again, and so on in continua- tion.

209. The second file will aim, at the instant the first brings down pieces to re-load, and will conform in all respects to that which has just been prescribed for the first file.

210. Alter the first fire, the front and rear rank men will not be required to fire at the same time.

211. Each man after loading, will return to the position of ready and continue the fire.

212. When the instructor wishes the fire to cease, he will command.

### Cease—FIRING.

213. At this command the men will cease firing. If they have fired, they will load their pieces and bring them to a shoulder; if at the position of *ready*, they will half-cock and shoulder arms. If in the position of *aim*, they will bring down their pieces, half- cock, and shoulder arms.

### To fire by rank.

214. The fire by rank will be executed by each entire rank, al- ternately.

215. The instructor will command :

1. *Fire by rank.* 2. *Squad.* 3. READY. 4. *Rear rank.* 5. AIM. 6. FIRE. 7. LOAD.

216. At the third command, the two ranks will take the posi- tion of *ready*, as prescribed in the direct fire.

217. At the seventh command, the rear rank will execute that which has been prescribed in the direct fire, and afterwards take the position of *ready*.

218. As soon as the instructor sees several men of the rear rank in the position of ready, he will command :

1. *Front rank.* 2. AIM. 3. FIRE. 4. LOAD.

219. At these commands, the men in the front rank will execute what has been prescribed for the rear rank, but they will not step off with the right foot.

220. The instructor will recommence the firing by the rear rank, and will thus continue to alternate from rank to rank, until he shall wish the firing to cease, when he will command, *cease firing*, which will be executed as heretofore prescribed.

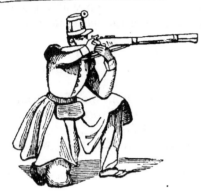

## LESSON V.

### *To fire and load kneeling.*

221. In this exercise the squad will be supposed loaded and drawn up in one rank. The instruction will be given to each man individually, without times or motions, and in the following manner.

222. The instructor will command:

### FIRE AND LOAD KNEELING

223. At this command, the man on the right of the squad will move forward three paces and halt; then carry the right foot to the rear and to the right of the left heel, and in a position convenient for placing the right knee upon the ground in bending the left leg; place the right knee upon the ground; lower the piece, the left fore arm supported upon the thigh on the same side, the right hand on the small of the stock, the butt resting on the right thigh, the left hand supporting the piece near the lower band

224 He will next move the right leg to the left around the knee supported on the ground, until this leg is nearly perpendicular to the direction of the left foot, and thus seat himself comfortably on the right heel.

225. Raise the piece with the right hand and support it with the left, holding it near the lower band, the left elbow resting on the lef thigh near the knee; seize the hammer with the thumb, the fore-finger under the guard; cock and seize the piece at the small of the stock; bring the piece to the shoulder, *aim* and *fire.*

226 Bring the piece down, as soon as it is fired, and support it with the left hand, the butt resting on the right thigh; carry the piece to the rear, rising on the knee, the barrel downwards, the butt resting on the ground; in this position support the piece with the left hand at the upper band, draw cartridge with the right and load the piece, ramming the ball, if necessary, with both hands.

226. When loaded, bring the piece to the front with the left hand, which holds it at the upper band; seize it at the same time with the right hand at the small of the stock; turn the piece, the barrel uppermost and nearly horizontal, the left elbow resting on the left thigh; half-cock, remove the old cap and prime, rise, and return to the ranks.

228. The second man will then be taught what has just been prescribed for the first, and so on through the remainder of the squad.

### *To fire and load lying.*

229. In this exercise the squad will be in one rank and loaded; v.

the instruction will be given individually and without times or motions.

230. The instructor will command :

FIRE AND LOAD LYING.

231. At this command, the man on the right of the squad will move forward three paces and halt ; he will then bring his piece to an order, drop on both knees, and place himself on the ground flat on his belly. In this position he will support the piece nearly horizontal with the left hand, holding it near the lower band, the butt end of the piece and the left elbow resting on the ground, the barrel uppermost ; cock the piece with the right hand, and carry this hand to the small of the stock ; raise the piece with both hands, press the butt against the shoulder, and resting on both elbows, *aim* and *fire*.

232. As soon as he has fired, bring the piece down and turn upon his left side, still resting on his left elbow ; bring back the piece until the cock is opposite his breast, the butt end resting on the ground ; take out a cartridge with the right hand ; seize the small of the stock with this hand, holding the cartridge with the thumb and two first fingers ; he will then throw himself on his back, still holding the piece with both hands ; carry the piece to the rear, place the butt between the heels, the barrel up, the muzzle elevated. In this position, charge cartridge, draw rammer, ram cartridge, and return rammer.

233. When finished loading, the man will turn again upon his left side, remove the old cap and prime, then raise the piece vertically, rise, turn about, and resume his position in the ranks.

234. The second man will be taught what has just been prescribed for the first, and so on throughout the squad.

LESSON VI.—*Bayonet Exercise.*

235. The bayonet exercise in this book will be confined to two movements, the *guard against infantry*, and the *guard against cavalry*. The men will be placed in one rank, with two paces interval, and being at shoulder arms the instructor will command :

1. *Guard against Infantry.*
2. GUARD.

One time and two motions.

236. (*First motion.*) Make a half face to the right, turning on both heels, the

feet square to each other; at the same time raise the piece slightly, and seize it with the left hand above and near the lower band.

237. (*Second motion.*) Carry the right foot twenty inches perpendicularly to the rear, the right heel on the prolongation of the left, the knees slightly bent, the weight of the body resting equally on both legs; lower the piece with both hands, the barrel uppermost, the left elbow against the body; seize the piece at the same time with the right hand at the small of the stock, the arms falling naturally, the point of the bayonet slightly elevated.

### Shoulder—Arms.

#### One time and one motion.

238. Throw up the piece with the left hand, and place it against the right shoulder, at the same time bring the right heel by the side of the left and face to the front.

### 1. *Guard against Cavalry.* 2. Guard.

#### One time and two motions.

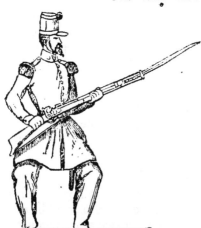

239. Both motions the same as for *guard against infantry,* except that the right hand will be supported against the hip, and the bayonet held at the height of the eye, as in *charge bayonet.*

### Shoulder—Arms.

#### One time and one motion.

240. Spring up the piece with the left hand and place it against the right shoulder, at the same time bring the right heel by the side of the left, and face to the front.

### PART THIRD.

241. When the recruits are well established in the *principles and mechanism of the step, the position of the body, and the manual of arms,* the instructor will unite eight men, at least, and twelve men, at most, in order to teach them the principles of alignment, the principles of the touch of elbows in marching to the front, the principles of the march by the flank, wheeling from a halt, wheeling in marching, and the change of direction to the side of the guide. He will place the squad in one rank elbow to elbow, and number them from right to left.

## Lesson I.

### *Alignments.*

242. The instructor will at first teach the recruits to align themselves man by man, in order the better to make them comprehend the principles of alignment; to this end, he will command the two men on the right flank to march two paces to the front, and having aligned them, he will caution the remainder of the squad to move up, as they may be successively called, each by his number, and align themselves successively on the line of the first two men.

243. Each recruit, as designated by his number, will turn the head and eyes to the right as prescribed in the first lesson of the first part, and will march in *quick time two paces forward*, shortening the last, so as to find himself about six inches behind the new alignment, which he ought never to pass: he will next move up steadily by steps of two or three inches, the hams extended, to the side of the man next to him on the alignment, so that, without deranging the head, the line of the eyes, or that of the shoulders, he may find himself in the exact line of his neighbor, whose elbow he will lightly touch without opening his own.

244. The instructor seeing the rank well aligned, will command:

#### Front.

245. At this, the recruits will turn eyes to the front, and remain firm.

246. Alignments to the left will be executed on the same principles.

247. When the recruits shall have thus learned to align themselves man by man, correctly, and without groping or jostling, the instructor will cause the entire rank to align itself at once by the command:

#### *Right* (or *left*)—Dress.

248. At this, the rank, except the two men placed in advance, as a basis of alignment, will move up in *quick time*, and place themselves on the new line, according to the principles prescribed No. 243.

249. The instructor, placed five or six paces in front, and facing the rank, will carefully observe that the principles are followed, and then pass to the flank that has served as the basis to verify the alignment.

250. The instructor seeing the greater number of the rank aligned, will command—

#### Front.

251. The instructor may afterwards order *this* or *that* file *for-*

*To march to the front.*

256. The rank being correctly aligned, when the instructor shall wish to cause it to march by the front, he will place a well instructed man on the right or the left, according to the side on which he may wish the guide to be, and command—

1. *Squad, forward.* 2. *Guide right* (or *left.*) 3. MARCH.

, . 257. At the command *march*, the rank will step off smartly with the left foot; the guide will take care to march straight to the front, keeping his shoulders always in a square with that line.

258. The instructor will observe, in marching to the front, that the men touch lightly the elbow towards the side of the guide;

*ward* or *back*, designating each by its number. The file or files designated, only, will slightly turn the head towards the basis, to judge how much they ought to move up or back, steadily place themselves on the line, and then turn eyes to the front, without a particular command to that effect.

252. Alignments to the rear will be executed on the same principles, the recruits stepping back a little beyond the line, and then dressing up according to the principles prescribed No 243, the instructor commanding:

*Right* (or *left*) *backward*—DRESS.

253. After each alignment, the instructor will examine the position of the men, and cause the rank to come to *ordered arms*, to prevent too much fatigue, and also the danger of negligence at *shouldered arms*.

LESSON II.

254. The men having learned, in the first and second parts, to march with steadiness in common time, and to take steps equal in length and swiftness, will be exercised in the third part only in *quick time, double quick time* and the *run*: the instructor will cause them to execute successively, at these different gaits, the march to the front, the facing about in marching, the march by the flank, the wheels at a halt and in marching, and the changes of direction to the side of the guide.

. 255. The instructor will inform the recruits that at the command *march*, they will always move off in *quick time*, unless this command should be preceded by that of *double quick*.

*To march to the front.*

256. The rank being correctly aligned, when the instructor

shall wish to cause it to march by the front, he will place a
well instructed man on the right or the left, according to the
side on which he may wish the guide to be, and command :

1. *Squad, forward.*  2. *Guide right,* (or *left.*  3. MARCH.

257. At the command *march,* the rank will step off smartly
with the left foot; the guide will take care to march straight to
the front, keeping his shoulders always in a square with that
line.

258. The instructor will observe,in marching to the front,that
the men touch lightly the elbow towards the side of the guide ;
that they do not open out the left elbow, nor the right arm; that
they yield to pressure coming from the side of the guide, and resist that coming from the opposite side ; that they recover by insensible degrees the slight touch of the elbow, if lost; that they
maintain the head direct to the front, no matter on which side the
guide may be ; and if found before or behind the alignment, that
the man in fault corrects himself by shortening or lengthening
the step, by degrees, almost insensible.

259. The instructor will labor to cause recruits to comprehend
that the alignment can only be preserved, in marching, by the
regularity of the step, the touch of the elbow, and the mainte-
nance of the shoulders in a square with the line of direction ;
that if, for example, the step of some be longer than that of others,
or if some march faster than others, a separation of elbows, and
a loss of the alignment, would be inevitable ; that i (it being required that the head should be direct to the front) they do not
strictly observe the touch of elbows, it would be impossible for an
individual to judge whether he marches abreast with his neighbor,
or not, and whether there be not an interval between them.

260. The impulsion of the quick step having a tendency to
make men too easy and free in their movements, the instructor
will be careful to regulate the cadence of this step, and to habituate them to preserve always the erectness of the body, and the
due length of the pace

261. The men being well established in the principles of the
direct march, the instructor will exercise them in marching obliquely. The rank being in march, the instructor will command:

1. *Right* (or *left*) *oblique.*  2. MARCH.

262. At the second command, each man will make a half face
to the right (or left.) and will then march straight forward in the
new direction. As the men no longer touch elbows they will
glance along the shoulders of the nearest files. towards the side
to which they are obliquing, and will regulate their steps so that
the shoulders shall always be behind that of their next neighbor
on that side, and that his head shall conceal the heads of the other

men in the rank. Besides this, the men should preserve the same length of pace, and the same degree of obliquity.

263. The instructor wishing to resume the primitive direction, will command—

1. *Forward.*   2. MARCH.

264. At the second command, each man will make a half face to the left (or right) and all will then march straight to the front, conforming to the principles of the direct march.

*To march to the front in double quick time.*

265. When the several principles, heretofore explained, have become familiar to the recruits, and they shall be well established in the position of the body, the bearing of arms, and the mechan- ism, length, and swiftness of the step, the instructor will pass them from *quick* to *double quick* time, and the reverse, observing not to make them march obliquely in double quick time, till they are well established in the cadence of the step.

266. The squad being at a march in quick time, the instructor will command—

1. *Double quick.*   2. MARCH.

267. At the command *march*, which will be given when either foot is coming to the ground, the squad will step off in double quick time. The men will endeavor to follow the principles laid down in the first part of this book, and to preserve the alignment.

268. When the instructor wishes the squad to resume the step in quick time, he will command—

1. *Quick time.*   2. MARCH.

269. At the command *march*, which will be given when either foot is coming to the ground, the squad will retake the step in quick time.

270. The squad being in march, the instructor will halt it by the commands and means prescribed Nos. 29 and 30. The com- mand *halt*, will be given an instant before the foot is ready to be placed on the ground.

271. The squad being in march in double quick time, the in- structor will occasionally cause it to mark time by the commands prescribed No. 171. The men will then mark double quick time, without altering the cadence of the step. He will also cause them to pass from the direct to the oblique step, and reciprocally, conforming to what has been prescribed No. 261, and following.

272. The squad being at a halt, the instructor will cause it to march in double quick time, by preceding the command *march*, by *double quick.*

273. The instructor will endeavor to regulate well the cadence of this step.

*To face about in marching.*

274. If the squad be marching in quick, or double quick time, and the instructor should wish to march it in retreat, he will command—

1. *Squad right about.* 2. MARCH.

275. At the command *march*, which will be given at the instant the left foot is coming to the ground, the recruit will bring this foot to the ground, and turning on it, will face to the rear; he will then place the right foot in the new direction, and step off with the left foot.

*To march backwards.*

276. The squad being at a halt, if the instructor should wish to march it in the back step, he will command:

1. *Squad backward.* 2. *Guide left* (or *right.*) 3. MARCH.

277. The back step will be executed by the means prescribed No. 178.

278. The instructor, in this step, will be watchful that the men do not lean on each other.

279. As the march to the front in quick time should only be executed at shouldered arms, the instructor, in order not to fatigue the men too much, and also to prevent negligence in gait and position, will halt the squad from time to time, and cause arms to be ordered.

280. In marching at *double quick time*, the men will always carry their pieces on the *right shoulder,* or at a *trail. This rule is general.*

281. If the instructor shall wish the pieces carried at a trail, he will give the command *trail arms*, before the command *double quick.* If, on the contrary, this command be not given, the men will shift their pieces to the right shoulder at the command *double quick.* In either case, at the command *halt*, the men will bring their pieces to the position of *shoulder arms. This rule is general.*

## LESSON III.

*To march by the flank.*

282. The rank being at a halt, and correctly aligned, the instructor will command—

I. *Squad, right*—FACE. 2. *Forward.* 3. MARCH.

283. At the last part of the first command, the rank will face to the right; the even numbered men, after facing to the right, will step quickly to the right side of the odd numbered men, the

latter standing fast, so that when the movement is executed, the men will be formed into files of two men abreast.

284. At the third command, the squad will step off smartly with the left foot ; the files keeping aligned, and preserving their intervals.

285. The march by the left flank will be executed by the same commands, substituting the word *left* for *right*, and by inverse means ; in this case, the even numbered me ., after facing to the left, will stand fast, and the odd numbered will place themselves on their left.

286. The instructor will place a well instructed soldier by the side of the recruit who is at the head of the rank, to regulate the step, and to conduct him ; and it will be enjoined on this recruit to march always elbow to elbow with the soldier.

287. The instructor will cause to be observed in the march, by the flank, the following rules :

*That the step be executed according to the principles prescribed for the direct step ;*

Because these principles, without which, men placed elbow to elbow, in the same rank, cannot preserve unity and harmony of movement, are of a more necessary observance in marching in file.

*That the head of the man who immediately precedes, covers the heads of all who are in front ;*

Because it is the most certain rule by which each man may maintain himself in the exact line of the file.

288. The instructor will place himself habitually five or six paces on the flank of the rank marching in file, to watch over the execution of the principles prescribed above.  He will also place himself sometimes in its rear, halt, and suffer it to pass fifteen or twenty paces, the better to see whether the men cover each other accurately.

289. When he shall wish to halt the rank, marching by the flank, and to cause it to face to the front, he will command :

1. *Squad.* 2. Halt. 3. Front.

290. At the second command, the rank will halt, and afterwards no man will stir, although he may have lost his distance. This prohibition is necessary, to habituate the men to a constant preservation of their distances.

291. At the third command, each man will front by facing to the left, if marching by the right flank, and by a face to the right, if marching by the left flank.  The rear rank men will at the same time move quickly into their places, so as to form the squad again into one rank.

292. When the men have become accustomed to marching by the flank, the instructor will cause them to change direction by file ; for this purpose, he will command :

1. *By left file* (or *right.*) 2. MARCH.

293. At the command *march,* the first file will change direction to the left (or right) in describing a small arc of a circle, and will then march straight forward; the two men of this file, in wheeling, will keep up the touch of the elbows, and the man on the side to which the wheel is made, will shorten the first three or four steps. Each file will come successively to wheel on the same spot where that which preceded it wheeled.

294. The instructor will also cause the squad to face by the right or left flank in marching, and for this purpose will command :

1. *Squad by the right* (or *left*) *flank.* 2. MARCH.

395. At the second command, which will be given a little before either foot comes to the ground, the recruits will turn the body, plant the foot that is raised in the new direction, and step off with the other foot without altering the cadence of the step: the men will double or undouble rapidly.

296. If, in facing by the right or the left flank, the squad should face to the rear, the men will come into one rank, agreeably to the principles indicated No. 291. It is to be remarked that it is the men who are in rear who always move up to form into single rank, and in such manner as never to invert the order of the numbers in the rank.

297. If, when the squad has been faced to the rear, the instructor should cause it to face by the left flank, it is the even numbers who will double by moving to the left of the odd numbers ; but if by the right flank, it is the odd numbers who will double to the right of the even numbers.

298. This lesson, like the preceding one, will be practised with pieces at a shoulder ; but the instructor may, to give relief by change, occasionally order *support arms,* and he will require of the recruits marching in this position, as much regularity as in the former.

*To march by the flank in double quick time.*

299. The principles of the march by the flank in double quick time, are the same as in quick time. The instructor will give the commands prescribed No. 282, taking care always to give the command *double quick* before that of *march.*

300. He will pay the greatest attention to the cadence of the step.

301. The instructor will cause the change of direction, and the

march by the flank, to be executed in double quick time, by the same commands, and according to the same principles, as in quick time.

302. The instructor will cause the pieces to be carried either on the *right shoulder* or at a *trail*.

303. The instructor will sometimes march the squad by the flank, without doubling the files.

304. The principles of this march are the same as in two ranks, and it will always be executed in quick time.

305. The instructor will give the commands prescribed No. 282, but he will be careful to caution the squad not to double files.

306. The instructor will be watchful that the men do not bend their knees unequally, which would cause them to tread on the heels of the men in front, and also to lose the cadence of the step and their distances.

307. The various movements in this lesson will be executed in single rank. In the changes of direction, the leading man will change direction without altering the length or the cadence of the step. The instructor will recall to the attention of the men, that in facing by the right or left flank in marching, they will no double, qut march in one rank.

LESSON IV.

WHEELINGS.

*General Principles of Wheeling.*

308. Wheelings are of two kinds: from halts, or on fixed pivots, and in march, or on moveable pivots.

309. Wheeling on a fixed pivot takes place in passing a corps from the order in battle to the order in column, or from the latter to the former.

310. Wheels in marching take place in changes of direction in column, as often as this movement is executed to the side opposite to the guide.

311. In wheels from a halt, the pivot man only turns in his place, without advancing or receding.

312. In the wheels in marching, the pivot takes steps of nine or eleven inches, according as the squad is marching in quick or double quick time, so as to clear the wheeling point, which is necessary, in order that the subdivisions of a column may change direction without losing their distances, as will be explained in the school of the company.

313. The man on the wheeling flank will take the full step of twenty-eight inches, or thirty-three inches, according to the gait.

*Wheeling from a halt, or ,on a fixed pivot.*

314. The rank being at a halt, the instructor will place a well instructed man on the wheeling flank to conduct it, and then command :

1. *By squad, right wheel.* 2 MARCH.

315. At the second command, the rank will step off with the left foot, turning at the same time the head a little to the left, the eyes fixed on the line of the eyes of the men to their left; the pivot-man will merely mark time in gradually turning his body, in order to conform himself to the movement of the marching flank; the man who conducts this flank will take steps of twenty-eight inches, and from the first step advance a little the left shoulder, cast his eyes from time to time along the rank and feel constantly the elbow of the next man lightly, but never push him.

316. The other men will feel lightly the elbow of the next man towards the pivot, resist pressure coming from the opposite side, and each will conform himself to the marching flank—shortening his step according to his approximation to the pivot.

217. The instructor will make the rank wheel round the circle once or twice before halting, in order to cause the principles to be the better understood, and he will be watchful that the centre does not break.

318. He will cause the wheel to the left to be executed according to the same principles.

319. When the instructor shall wish to arrest the wheel, he will command :

1. *Squad.* 2. HALT.

320. At the second command, the rank will halt, and no man stir. The instructor, going to the flank opposite the pivot, will place the two outer men of that flank in the direction he may wish to give to the rank, without however displacing the pivot, who will conform the line of his shoulders to this direction. The instructor will take care to have between these two men, and the pivot, only the space necessary to contain the other men. He will then command :

*Left* (or *right*)—DRESS.

321. At this, the rank will place itself on the alignment of the two men established as the basis, in conformity with the principles prescribed.

322. The instructor will next command FRONT, which will be executed as prescribed No. 245.

*Remarks on the principles of the wheel from a halt.*

323. Turn a little the head towards the marching flank, and fix.

the eyes on the line of the eyes of the men who are on that side;

Because, otherwise, it would be impossible for each man to regulate the length of his step so as to conform his own movement to that of the marching flank.

*Touch lightly the elbow of the next man towards the pivot;*

In order that the files may not open out in the wheel.

*Resist pressure that comes from the side of the marching flank;*

Because, if this principle be neglected, the pivet, which ought to be a fixed point, in wheels from a halt, might be pushed out of its place by pressure.

*Wheeling in marching, or on a moveable pivot.*

324. When the recruits have been brought to execute well the wheel from a halt, they will be taught to wheel in marching.

325. To this end, the rank being in march, when the instructor shall wish to cause it to change direction to the reverse flank, (to the side opposite to the guide or pivot flank,) he will command:

1. *Right* (or *left*) *wheel.* 2 MARCH.

326. The first command will be given when the rank is yet *four* paces from the wheeling point.

327. At the second command, the wheel will be executed in the same manner as from a halt, except that the touch of the elbow will remain towards the marching flank (or side of the guide) instead of the side of the actual pivot; that the pivot man, instead of merely turning in his place, will conform himself to the movement of the marching flank, feel lightly the elbow of the next man, take steps of full nine inches, and thus gain ground forward in describing a small curve so as to clear the point of the wheel. The middle of the rank will bend slightly to the rear. As soon as the movement shall commence, the man who conducts the marching flank will cast his eyes on the ground over which he will have to pass.

328. The wheel being ended the instructor will command:

1. *Forward.* 2. MARCH.

339. The first command will be pronounced when *four* paces are yet required to complete the change of direction.

330. At the command *march*, which will be given at the instant of completing the wheel, the man who conducts the march-

ing flank will direct himself straight forward; the pivot man and all the rank will retake the step of twenty-eight inches, and bring the head direct to the front.

*Turning, or change of direction to the side of the guide.*

331. The change of direction to the side of the guide, in march-ing, will be executed as follows : The instructor will command :

1. *Left* (or right) *turn.* 2. MARCH.

332. The first command will be given when the rank is yet four paces from the turning point.

333. At the command *march*, to be pronounced at the instant the rank ought to turn, the guide will face to the left (or right) in marching, and move forward in the new direction without short-ening or quickening the cadence, and without shortening or lengthening the step. The whole rank will promptly conform itself to the new direction ; to effect which, each man will ad-vance the shoulder opposite to the guide, take the double quick step, to carry himself in the new direction, turn the head and eyes to the side of the guide, and retake the touch of the elbow on that side, in placing himself on the alignment of the guide, from whom he will take the step, and then resume the direct po-sition of the head. Each man will thus arrive successively on the alignment.

*Wheeling and changing direction to the side of the guide, in double quick time.*

334. When the recruits comprehend and execute well, in quick time, the wheels at a halt and in marching, and the change of direction to the side of the guide, the instructor will cause the same movements to be repeated in double quick time.

335. These various movements will be executed by the same commands and according to the same principles as in quick time, except that, the command *double quick* will precede that of *march*. In wheeling while marching, the pivot man will take steps of eleven inches, and in the changes of direction to the side of the guide, the men on the side opposite the guide must increase the gait in order to bring themselves in line.

336. The instructor, in order not to fatigue the recruits, and not to divide their attention will cause them to execute the seve-ral movements of which this lesson is composed, first without arms, and next, after the mechanism be well comprehended, with arms.

LESSON V.

*Long marches in double quick time and the run.*

337. The instructor will cause to be resumed the exercises in double quick time and the run, with arms and knapsacks.

338. He will cause long marches to be executed in double quick time, both by the front and by the flank, and by constant practice will lead the men to pass over a distance of five miles in sixty minutes. The pieces will be carried on either shoulder, and sometimes at a trail.

339. He will also exercise them in long marches at a run, the pieces carried at will; the men will be instructed to keep as united as possible, without however exacting much regularity, which is impracticable.

340. The run, in actual service, will only be resorted to when it may be highly important to reach a given point with great promptitude.

*To stack arms.*

The men being at order arms, the instructor will command:

*Stack*—ARMS.

341. At this command, the front rank man of every even numbered file will pass his piece before him, seizing it with the left hand near the upper band; will place the butt a little in advance of his left toe, the barrel turned towards the body, and draw the rammer slightly from its place; the front rank man of every odd numbered file will also draw the rammer slightly, and pass his piece to the man next on his left, who will seize it with the right hand near the upper band, and place the butt a little in advance of the right toe of the man next on his right, the barrel turned to the front; he will then cross the rammers of the two pieces, the rammer of the piece of the odd numbered man being inside ; the rear rank man of every even file will also draw his rammer, lean his piece forward, the lock-plate downwards, advance the right foot about six inches, and insert the rammer between the rammer and barrel of the piece of his front rank man ; with his left hand he will place the butt of his piece on the ground, thirty-two inches in rear of, and perpendicular to, the front rank, bringing back his right foot by the side of the left; the front rank man of every even file will at the same time lean the stack to the rear, quit it with his right hand and force the rammers down. The stack being thus formed, the rear rank men of every odd file will pass his piece into his left hand, the barrel to the front and inclining it forward, will rest it on the stack.

342. The men of both ranks having taken the position of the soldier without arms, the instructor will command :

1. *Break ranks.* 2. MARCH.

*To resume arms.*

343. Both ranks being re-formed in rear of their stacks, the instructor will command :

*Take*—ARMS.

**344.** At this command, the rear rank man of every odd numbered file will withdraw his piece from the stack ; the front rank man of every even file will seize his own piece with the left hand and that of the man on his right with his right hand, both above the lower band ; the rear rank man of the even file will seize his piece with the right hand below the lower band ; these two men will raise up the stack to loosen the rammers; the front rank man of every odd file will facilitate the disengagement of the rammers, if necessary, by drawing them out slightly with the left hand, and will receive his piece from the hand of the man next on his left; the four men will retake the position of the soldier at order arms.

END OF THE SCHOOL OF THE SOLDIER.

# TITLE THIRD.

## SCHOOL OF THE COMPANY.

*General Rules and division of the School of the Company.*

1. Instruction by company will always precede that by battalion, and the object being to prepare the soldiers for the higher school, the exercises of detail by company will be strictly adhered to, as well in respect to principles, as the order of progression herein prescribed.

2. There will be attached to a company undergoing elementary instruction, a captain, a covering sergeant, and a certain number of file closers, the whole posted in the manner indicated, Title First, and, according to the same title, the officer charged with the exercise of such company will herein be denominated the *instructor.*

3. The School of the Company will be divided into six lessons, and each lesson will comprehend five articles, as follows—

### LESSON I.

1. To open ranks.
2. Alignments in open ranks.
3. Manual of arms.
4. To close ranks.
5. Alignments, and manual of arms in closed ranks.

### LESSON II.

1. To load in four times and at will.
2. To fire by company.
3. To fire by file.
4. To fire by rank.
5. To fire by the rear rank.

### LESSON III.

1. To march in line of battle.
2. To halt the company marching in line of battle, and to align it.
3. Oblique march in line of battle.
4. To mark time, to march in double quick time, and the back step.
5. To march in retreat in line of battle.

## Lesson IV.

1. To march by the flank.
2. To change direction by file.
3. To halt the company marching by the flank, and to face it to the front.
4. The company being in march by the flank, to form it on the right or left by file into line of battle.
5. The company marching by the flank, to form it by company or platoon into line, and cause it to face to the right and left in marching.

## Lesson V.

1. To break into column by platoon either at a halt, or while marching.
2. To march in column.
3. To change direction.
4. To halt the column.
5. Being in column by platoon, to form to the right or left into line of battle, either at a halt or marching.

## Lesson VI.

1. To break into platoons, and to re-form the company.
2. To break files to the rear, and to cause them to re-enter into line.
3. To march in column *in route*, and to execute the movements incident thereto.
4. Countermarch.
5. Being in column by platoon, to form on the right or left into line of battle.

4. The company will always be formed in two ranks. The instructor will then cause the files to be numbered, and for this purpose will command—

*In each rank*—Coun: Twos.

5. At this command, the men count in each rank, from right to left, pronouncing in a loud and distinct voice, in the same tone, without hurry and without turning the head, *one, two*, according to the place which each one occupies. He will also cause the company to be divided into platoons and sections, taking care that the first platoon is always composed of an even number of files.
6. The instructor will be as clear and concise as possible in his explanations; he will cause faults of detail to be rectified by the captain, to whom he will indicate them, if the captain should not have himself observed them; and the instructor will not otherwise

interfere, unless the captain should not well comprehend, or should badly execute his intentions.

7. Composure, or presence of mind, in him who commands, and in those who obey, being the first means of órder in a body of troops, the instructor will labor to habituate the company to this essential quality, and will himself give the example.

## LESSON FIRST.
### ARTICLE FIRST.
### *To open ranks.*

8. The company being at ordered arms, the ranks and file closers well aligned, when the instructor shall wish to cause the ranks to be opened, he will direct the left guide to place himself on the left of the front rank, which being executed, he will command—

1. *Attention*   2. *Company.*   3. *Shoulder*—ARMS.   4. *To the rear open order.*

9. At the fourth command, the covering sergeant, and the left guide, will step of smartly to the rear, four paces from the front rank, in order to mark the alignment of the rear rank. They will judge this distance by the eye, without counting the steps.

10. The instructor will place himself at the same time on the right flank, in order to observe, if these two non commissioned officers are on a line parallel to the front rank, and it necessary, to correct their positions, which being executed, he will command:

### 5. MARCH.

11. At this command, the front rank will stand fast.

12. The rear rank will step to the rear, without counting the steps, and will place themselves on the alignment marked for this rank, conforming to what is prescribed in the school of the soldier, No. 252.

13. The covering sergeant will align the rear rank on the left guide placed to mark the left of this rank.

14. The file closers will march to the rear at the same time with the rear rank, and will place themselves two paces from this rank when it is aligned.

15. The instructor seeing the rear rank aligned, will command :

### 6. FRONT.

16. At this command, the sergeant on the left of the rear rank will turn to his place as a file closer.

17. The rear rank being aligned, the instructor will direct the

captain and the covering sergeant to observe the men in their
respective ranks, and to correct if necessary, the positions of per·
sons and pieces.

### Article Second.

*Alignments in open ranks.*

18. The ranks being open, the instructor will, in the first exercises, align the ranks, man by man, the better to inculcate the
principles.
19. To effect this, he will cause two or four men on the right
or left of each rank to march two or three paces forward, and,
after having aligned them, command :

. *By file right* (or *left*)—Dress.

20. At this, the men of each rank will move up successively
on the alignment each man being preceded by his neighbor in
the same rank, towards the basis, by two paces, and having correctly aligned himself, will cast his eyes to the front.
21. Successive alignments having habituated the soldiers to
dress correctly, the instructor will cause the ranks to align themselves at once, forward and backward, sometimes in a direction
parallel, and sometimes in one oblique, to the original direction,
giving, in each case, two or four men to serve as a basis of align· ·
ment to each rank.   To effect which, he will command :

1. *Right* (or *left*)—Dress.   2. Front.
or
1. *Right* (or *left*) *backward*—Dress.   2. Front.

22. In oblique alignments, in *opened* ranks, the men of the
rear rank will not seek to cover their file leaders, as the sole ob·
ject of the exercise is to teach them to align themselves correctly
in their respective ranks, in the different directions.
23. In the several alignments, the captain will superintend the
front rank, and the covering sergeant the rear rank.   For this
purpose, they will place themselves on the side by which the
ranks are dressed.
24. In oblique alignments, the men will conform the line of
their shoulders to the new direction of their rank, and will place
themselves on the alignments as has been prescribed in the school
of the soldier, No. 248 or No. 252, according as the new direction shall be in front or rear of the original one.
25. At the end of each alignment, the captain and the cover·
ing sergeant will pass along the front of the ranks to correct the
position of persons and arms.

ARTICLE THIRD.

*Manual of arms.*

26. The ranks being open, the instructor will place himself in a position to see the ranks, and will command the manual of arms in the following order :

| | |
|---|---|
| *Present arms.* | *Shoulder arms.* |
| *Order arms.* | |
| *Ground arms.* | |
| *Raise arms.* | *Shoulder arms.* |
| *Support arms.* | *Shoulder arms.* |
| *Fix bayonet.* | *Shoulder arms.* |
| *Charge bayonet.* | *Shoulder arms.* |
| *Trail arms.* | *Shoulder arms.* |
| *Unfix bayonet.* | *Shoulder arms.* |
| *Secure arms.* | *Shoulder arms.* |

*Load in nine times.*

27. The instructor will take care that the position of the body, of the feet, and of the piece, be always exact, and that the times be briskly executed and close to the person.

ARTICLE FOURTH.

*To close ranks.*

28. The manual of arms being ended, the instructor will command :

1. *Close order.* 2. MARCH.

29. At the command *march,* the rear rank will close up in quick time, each man directing himself on his file leader.

ARTICLE FIFTH.

*Alignments, and manual of arms in closed ranks.*

30. The ranks being closed, the instructor will cause to be executed parallel and oblique alignments by the right and left, forward and backward, observing to place always two or four files to serve as a basis of alignment. He will give the commands prescribed, No. 21.

31. In alignments in closed ranks, the captain will superintend the front rank, and the covering sergeant the rear rank. They will habituate themselves to judge the alignment by the lines of the eyes and shoulders, in casting a glance of the eye along the front and rear of the ranks.

32. The moment the captain perceives the greater number of the front rank aligned, he will command—FRONT, and rectify, afterwards, if necessary, the alignment of the other men by the means prescribed in the school of the soldier, No. 251. The rear rank will conform to the alignment of the front rank, superintended by the covering sergeant.

33. The ranks being steady, the instructor will place himself on the flank to verify the alignment. He will also see that each rear rank man covers accurately his file leader.

34. In oblique alignments, the instructor will observe what is prescribed, No. 24.

35. In all alignments, the file closers will preserve the distance of two paces from the rear rank.

36. The alignments being ended, the instructor will cause to be executed the manual of arms.

37. The instructor, wishing to rest the men, without deranging the alignment, will first cause arms to be supported, or ordered, and then command:

*In place*—REST.

38. At this command, the men will no longer be constrained to preserve silence or steadiness of position ; but they will always keep one or other heel on the alignment.

39. If on the contrary, the instructor should wish to rest the men without constraining them to preserve the alignment, he will command :

REST.

40. At which command, the men will not be required to preserve immobility, or to remain in their places.

41. The instructor may, also, when he shall judge proper, cause arms to be stacked, which will be executed as prescribed, school of the soldier·

## LESSON SECOND.

42. The instructor wishing to pass to the second lesson, will cause the company to take arms, if stacks have been formed, and command—

   1. *Attention.*  2. *Company.*  3. *Shoulder*—ARMS.

43. The instructor will then cause loadings and firings to be executed in the following order :

### ARTICLE FIRST.

*To load in four times and at will.*

44. Loading in four *times* will be commanded and executed as prescribed in the school of the soldier, No· 182, and following·

**The** instructor will cause this exercise to be often repeated, in succession, before passing to load at will.

45. Loading at will, will be commanded and executed as prescribed in the school of the soldier, No. 187. In priming when loading in four *times*, and also at will, the captain and covering sergeant will half face to the right with the men, and face to the front when the man next to them, respectively, brings his piece to the shoulder.

46. The instructor will labor to the utmost to cause the men, in the different loadings, to execute what has been prescribed in the school of the soldier, Nos. 188 and 189.

47. Loading at will, being that of battle, and consequently the one with which it is most important to render the men familiar, it will claim preference in the exercises the moment the men be well established in the principles. To these they will be brought by degrees, so that every man may be able to load with cartridges and to fire at least three rounds in a minute with ease and regularity.

### ARTICLE SECOND.

#### To fire by company.

48. The instructor, wishing to cause the fire by company to be executed, will command:

1. *Fire by company.* 2. *Commence firing.*

49. At the first command, the captain will promptly place himself opposite the centre of his company, and four paces in rear of the line of file closers; the covering sergeant will retire to that line, and place himself opposite to his interval. *This rule is general, for both the captain and covering sergeant, in all the different firings.*

50. At the second command, the captain will add: 1. Company; 2. READY; 3. AIM; 4. FIRE; 5. LOAD.

51. At the command *load*, the men will load their pieces, and then take the position of *ready*, as prescribed in the school of the soldier.

52. The captain will immediately recommence the firing, by the commands:

1. *Company.* 2. AIM. 3. FIRE. 4. LOAD.

53. The firing will be thus continued until the signal to cease firing is sounded.

54. The captain will sometimes cause aim to be taken to the right and left, simply observing to pronounce *right* (or *left*) *oblique,* before the command *aim.*

### Article Third.

### *The fire by file.*

55. The instructor wishing to cause the fire by file to be executed, will command :

1. *Fire by file.* 2. *Company.* 3. Ready. 4. *Commence firing.*

56. The third and fourth commands will be executed as prescribed in the school of the soldier, No. 206 and following.

57. The fire will be commenced by the right file of the company ; the next file will take aim at the instant the first brings
down pieces to re-load, and so on to the left ; but this progression
will only be observed in the first discharge, after which each man
will re-load and fire without regulating himself by others, conforming himself to what is prescribed in the school of the soldier,
No. 211.

### Article Fourth.

### *To fire by rank.*

58. The instructor wishing the fire by rank to be executed, will
command :

1. *Fire by rank.* 2. *Company.* 3. Ready. 4. *Rear rank*
Aim. 5. Fire. 6. Load.

59. The fifth and sixth commands will be executed as is prescribed in the school of the soldier, No. 216, and following.

60. When the instructor sees one or two pieces in the rear
rank at a ready, he will command :

1. *Front rank.* 2. Aim. 3. Fire. 4. Load.

61. The firing will be continued thus by alternate ranks, until
the signal is given to cease firing.

62. The instructor will sometimes cause aim to be taken to the
right and left, conforming to what is prescribed No. 54.

63. The instructor will cause the firing to cease, whether by
company, by file, or by rank, by sounding the signal to *cease firing,*
and at the instant this sound commences, the men will cease to
fire, conforming to what is prescribed in the school of the soldier,
No. 213.

64. The signal to cease firing will be always followed by a
bugle note ; at which sound, the captain and covering sergeant
will promptly resume their places in line, and will rectify, if necessary, the alignment of the ranks.

65. In this school, except when powder is used, the signal to cease firing will be indicated by the command *cease firing*, which will be pronounced by the instructor when he wishes the semblance of firing to cease.

66. The command *posts* will be likewise substituted, under similar circumstances, for the bugle note employed as the signal for the return of the captain and covering sergeant to their places in line, which command will be given when the instructor sees the men have brought their pieces to a shoulder.

67. The fire by file being that which is most frequently used against an enemy, it is highly important that it be rendered perfectly familiar to the troops. The instructor will, therefore, give it almost exclusive preference, and labor to cause the men to aim with care, and always, if possible, at some particular object. As it is of the utmost importance that the men should aim with precision in battle, this principle will be rigidly enforced in the exercises for purposes of instruction.

## ARTICLE FIFTH.

### To fire by the rear rank.

68. The instructor will cause the several fires to be executed to the rear, that is, by the rear rank. To effect this, he will command—

1. *Face by the rear rank.*   2. *Company.*   3. *About*—FACE.

69. At the first command, the captain will step out and place himself near to, and facing the right file of his company; the covering sergeant, and file closers, will pass quickly through the captain's interval, and place himself faced to the rear, the covering sergeant a pace behind the captain, and the file closers two paces from the front rank, opposite to their places in line, each passing behind the covering sergeant.

70. At the third command, which will be given at the instant the last file closer shall have passed through the interval, the company will face about; the captain will place himself in his interval in the rear rank, now become the front, and the covering sergeant will cover him in the front rank, now become the rear.

71. The company having faced by the rear rank, the instructor will cause it to execute the fire by company, both direct and oblique, the fire by file, and the fire by rank, by the commands and means prescribed in the three preceeding articles; the captain, covering sergeant, and the men will conform themselves, in like manner, to what is therein prescribed.

72. The fire by file, will commence on the left of the company, now become the right. In the fire by rank, the firing will commence with the front rank, now become the rear.

73. To resume the proper front, the instructor will command:

1. *Face by the front rank.* 2. *Company.* 3. *About*—FACE.

74. At the first command, the captain, covering sergeant and file closers, will conform to what is prescribed Nos. 69 and 70.

75. At the third command, the company having faced about, the captain and covering sergeant will resume their places in line.

76. In this lesson, the instructor will impress on the men the importance of aiming always at some particular object, and holding the piece as prescribed in the school of the soldier, No. 109.

77. The instructor will recommend to the captain to make a short pause between the command *aim* and *fire*, to give the men time to aim with accuracy.

78. The instructor will place himself in position to see the two ranks, in order to detect faults ; he will charge the captain and file closers to be equally watchful, and to report to him when the ranks are at rest.   He will remand, for individual instruction, the men who may be observed to load badly.

79. The instructor will recommend to the soldiers, in the firings, the highest degree of composure or presence of mind ; he will neglect nothing that may contribute to this end

80. He will give to the men, *as a general principle,* to maintain, in the direct fire, the left heel in its place, in order that the alignment of the ranks and files may not be deranged ; and he will verify, by examination, after each exercise in firing, the observance of this principle.

81. The instructor will observe, in addition to these remarks, all those which follow.

82. When the firing is executed with cartridges, it is particularly recommended that the men observe, in uncocking, whether smoke escapes from the tube, which is a certain indication that the piece has been discharged ; but if, on the contrary, no smoke escapes, the soldier, in such case, instead of re-loading, will pick and prime again.   If, believing the load to be discharged, the soldier should put a second cartridge in his piece, he ought, at least, to perceive it in ramming, by the height of the load ; and he would be very culpable, should he put in a third.   The instructor will always cause arms to be inspected after firing with cartridges, in order to observe if the fault has been committed, of putting three cartridges, without a discharge, in the same piece, in which case the ball screw will be applied.

83. It sometimes happens, when a cap has missed fire, that the tube is found stopped up with a hard, white, and compact powder; in this case, picking will be dispensed with, and a new cap substituted for the old one.

## LESSON THIRD.

### ARTICLE FIRST.

*To advance in a line of battle.*

84. The company being in a line of battle, and correctly aligned, when the instructor shall wish to exercise it in marching by the front, he will assure himself that the shoulders of the captain and covering sergeant are perfectly in the direction of their respective ranks, and that the sergeant accurately covers the captain ; the instructor will then place himself twenty-five or thirty paces in front of them, face to the rear, and place himself exactly on the prolongation of the line passing between their heels.

85. The instructor, being aligned on the directing file, will command :

### 1. *Company forward.*

86. At this, a sergeant, previously designated, will move six paces in advance of the captain ; the instructor, from the position prescribed, will correctly align this sergeant on the prolongation of the directing file.

87. This advance sergeant, whe is to be charged with the direction, will, the moment his position is assured, take two points on the ground, in the straight line which would pass between his own, and the heels of the instructor.

88. These dispositions being made, the instructor will step aside, and command :

### 2. MARCH.

89. At this, the company will step off with life. The directing sergeant will observe, with the greatest precision, the length and cadence of the step, marching on the two points he has chosen ; he will take in succession, and always a little before arriving at the point nearest to him, new points in advance, exactly in the same line with the first two, and at the distance of some fifteen or twenty paces from each other. The captain will march steadily in the trace of the directing sergeant, keeping always six paces from him ; the men will each maintian the head direct to the front, feel lightly the elbow of his neighbor on the side of direction, and conform himself to the principles prescribed, school of the soldier, for the march by the front.

90. The man next to the captain, will take special care not to pass him ; to this end, he will keep the line of his shoulders a little in the rear, but in the same direction with those of the captain.

91. The file closers will march at the habitual distance of two paces behind the rear rank.

92. If the men lose the step, the instructor will command :

*To the*—STEP.

93. At this command, the men will glance towards the direct-ing sergeant, retake the step from him, and again direct their eyes to the front.

94. The instructor will cause the captain and covering sergeant to be posted sometimes on the right, and sometimes on the left of the company.

95. The directing sergeant, in advance, having the greatest in-fluence on the march of the company, he will be selected for the precision of his step, his habit of maintaining his shoulders in a square or a given line of direction, and of prolonging that line without variation.

96. If this sergeant should fail to observe these principles, un-dulations in the front of the company must necessarily follow ; the men will be unable to contract the habit of taking steps equal in length and swiftness, and of maintaining their shoulders in a square with the line of direction—the only means of attaining perfection in the march in line.

97. The instructor, with a view the better to establish the men in the length and cadence of the step, and in the principles of the march in line, will cause the company to advance three or four hundred paces, at once, without halting, if the ground will permit. In the first exercises, he will march the company with open ranks, the better to observe the two ranks.

98. The instructor will see, with care, that all the principles of the march in line are strictly observed ; he will generally be on the directing flank, in a position to observe the two ranks, and the faults they may commit ; he will sometimes halt behind the directing file during some thirty successive steps, in order to judge whether the directing sergeant, or the directing file, deviate from the perpendicular.

ARTICLE SECOND.

*To halt the company, marching in line of battle, and to align it.*

99. The instructor, wishing to halt the company, will commmand :

1. *Company.* 2. HALT.

100. At the second command, the company will halt ; the di-recting sergeant will remain in advance, unless ordered to return to the line of file closers. The company being at a halt, the in-structor may advance the first three or four files on the side of di-

rection, and align the company on that basis, or he may confine himself to causing the alignment to be rectified. In this last case, he will command: *Captain, rectify the alignment.* The captain will direct the covering sergeant to attend to the rear rank, when each, glancing his eyes along his rank, will promptly rectify it, conforming to what is prescribed in the school of the soldier, No. 251.

### ARTICLE THIRD.

*Olique march in the line of battle.*

101. The company being in the direct march, when the instructor shall wish to cause it to march obliquely he will com. mand:

1. *Right* (or *left*) *oblique.* 2. MARCH.

102. At the command *march,* the company will take the oblique step. The men will accurately observe the principles prescribed in the school of the soldier, No. 262. The rear rank men will observe their distances, and march in rear of the man next on the right (or left) of their habitual file leaders.

103. When the instructor wishes the direct march to be re. sumed, he will command:

1. *Forward.* 2. MARCH·

'104· At the command *mach,* the company will resume the direct march. The instructor will move briskly twenty paces in front of the captain, and facing the company, will place himself exactly in the prolongation of the captain and covering sergeant; and then by a sign, will move the directing sergeant on the same line, if he be not already on it : the latter will immediately take two points on the ground between himself and the instructor, and as he advances, will take new points of direction, as is explained No. 89.

105. In the oblique march, the men not having the touch of elbows, the guide will always be on the side towards which the oblique is made, without any indication to that effect being given; and when the direct march is resumed, the guide will be, equally without indication, on the side where it was previous to the oblique:

106. The instructor will, at first, cause the oblique to be made towards the side of the guide. He will also direct the captain to have an eye on the directing sergeant, in order to keep on the same perpendicular line to the front with him, while following a parallel direction,

107. During the continuance of the march, the instructor will be watchful that the men follow parallel directions, in conforming to the principles prescribed in the school of the soldier, for pre-

serving the general alignment; whenever the men lose the alignment, he will be careful that they regain it by lengthening or
shortening the step, without altering the cadence, or changing the
direction.

108. The instructor will place himself in front of the company
and face to it, in order to regulate the march of the directing sergeant, or the man who is on the flank towards which the oblique
is made, and to see that the principles of the march are properly
observed, and that the files do not crowd.

### ARTICLE FOURTH.

*To mark time, to march in double quick time, and the back step.*

109. The company being in the direct march and in quick time'
the instructor, to cause it to mark time, will command :

1. Mark time.   2. MARCH.

110. To resume the march, he will command :

1. Forward.   2. MARCH.

111. To cause the march in double quick time, the instructor
will command :

1. Double quick.   2. MARCH.

112. The command *march* will be pronounced at the instant '
either foot is coming to the ground.

113. To resume quick time, the instructor will command—

1. Quick time.   2. MARCH.

114. The command *march* will be pronounced at the instant
either foot is coming to the ground.

115. The company being at a halt, the instructor may cause
it to march in the back step; to this effect, he will command :

1. Company backward.   2. MARCH.

116. The back step will be executed according to the principles prescribed in the school of the soldier No. 178, but the use of
it being rare, the instructor will not cause more than fifteen or
twenty steps to be taken in succession, and to that extent but sel-
dom.

117. The instructor ought not to exercise the company in marching in double quick time till the men are well established in the
length and swiftness of the pace in quick time: he will then endeavor to render the march of one hundred and seventy-five steps

in the minute equally easy and familiar, and also cause them to observe the same erectness of body and composure of mind, as if marching in quick time.

118. When marching in double quick time, if a subdivision (in a column) has to change direction by *turning*, or has to form into line, the men will quicken the pace to one hundred and eighty steps in a minute. The same swiftness of step will be observed uncer all circumstances where great rapidity of movement is required. But, as ranks of men cannot march any length of time at so swift a rate, without breaking or confusion, this acceleration will not be considered a prescribed exercise, and accordingly companies or battalions will only be habitually exercised in the double quick time of one hundred and sixty-five steps in the minute.

### Article Fifth.

*To march in retreat.*

119. The company being halted and correctly aligned, when the instructor shall wish to cause it to march in retreat, he will command—

1. *Company.*    2. *About*—Face.

120. The company having faced to the rear, the instructor will place himself in front of the directing file, conforming to what is prescribed, No. 84.

121. The instructor, being correctly established on the prolongation of the directing file, will command—

3. *Company forward.*

122. At this, the directing sergeant will conform himself to what is prescribed, Nos. 86 and 87, with this difference—he will place himself six paces in front of the line of file closers, now leading.

123. The covering sergeant will step into the line of file closers, opposite to his interval, and the captain will place himself in the rear rank, now become the front.

124. This disposition being promptly made, the instructor will command—

4. March.

125. At this, the directing sergeant, the captain, and the men, will conform themselves to what is prescribed No. 89, and following.

126. The instructor will cause to be executed, marching in retreat, all that is prescribed for marching in advance ; the commands and the means of execution will be the same.

5

127. The instructor having halted the company, will, when he may wish, cause it to face to the front by the commands 'prescribed No. 119. The captain, the covering sergeant, and the directing sergeant, will resume their habitual places in line, the moment they shall have faced about.

128. The company being in march by the front rank, if the instructor should wish it to march in retreat, he will cause the right about to be executed while marching, and to this effect will command—

1. *Company.* 2. *Right about.* 3. MARCH.

129. At the third command, the company will promptly face about, and recommence the march by the rear rank.

130. The directing sergeant will face about with the company, and will move rapidly six paces in front of the file closers, and upon the prolongation of the guide. The instructor will place him in the proper direction by the means prescribed No. 104. The captain, the covering sergeant, and the men, will conform to the principles prescribed for the march in retreat.

131. When the instructor wishes the company to march by the front rank, he will give the same commands, and will regulate the direction of the march by the same means.

132. The instructor will cause to be executed in double quick time, all the movements prescribed in the 3d, 4th, 5th, and 6th lessons of this school, with the exception of the march backwards, which will be executed only in quick time. He will give the same commands, observing to add *double quick* before the command *march.*

133. When the pieces are carried on the right shoulder, in quick time, the distance between the ranks will be sixteen inches. Whenever, therefore, the instructor brings the company from a shoulder to this position, the rear rank must shorten a little the first steps in order to gain the prescribed distance, and will lengthen the steps, on the contrary, in order to close up when the pieces are again brought to a shoulder. In marching in double quick time, the distance between the ranks will be twenty-six inches, and the pieces will be carried habitually on the right shoulder.

134. Whenever a company is halted, the men will bring their pieces at once to a shoulder at the command *halt.* The rear rank will close to its proper distance. *These rules are general.*

## LESSON FOURTH.

### ARTICLE FIRST.

*To march by the flank.*

135. The company being in line of battle, and at a halt, when

Some difficulty having been experienced in executing the move— ·
ments in Lesson IV, (page 67,) Col. Hardee was applied to for
information upon the subject. Subjoined is his answer.

In reply to your first question, I beg to say, that
if the Company be marching to the front and the command "By the right (or left) Flank" should be given,
the men double by fours in the same manner as when the
command "Right (or left) Face" is given at a halt.

Second point.—If the company be faced to the rear,
and the command 'Left (or right) Face" be given, No. 1
of the front rank faces at once and stands fast. No. 1 of
the rear rank steps one pace to the rear (his front) and at
the same time faces to the left. No. 2 of the front rank
faces and steps into the interval between the front rank
men; and No. 2 rear rank places himself on the extreme
right of the set of fours, thus :

$$\overline{\overline{2}} \quad \overline{\overline{1}} \quad \overline{\overline{2}} \quad \overline{\overline{1}} \quad \overline{\overline{2}} \quad \overline{\overline{1}} \quad \text{front rank,}$$

Faced to the rear $\overline{\overline{2}} \quad \overline{\overline{1}} \quad \overline{\overline{2}} \quad \overline{\overline{1}} \quad \overline{\overline{2}} \quad \overline{\overline{1}} \quad$ rear rank.

$$\| \quad \| \quad \|$$
$$\quad\quad 1 \quad 1$$

$$\| \quad \| \quad \|$$
Left face $\quad\quad\quad\quad 2$

$$\| \quad \| \quad \|$$
$$\quad\quad\quad\quad 1$$

$$\| \quad \| \quad \|$$
$$\quad\quad\quad\quad 2$$

The face to the right is made in the same manner except the movement is made on No. 2 front rank. The
front refered to is always the *real front*.

In Loading (p. 19) most of the instructors have
substituted the old system of placing the piece by the
side of the left foot, instead of between the feet.

the instructor shall wish to cause it to march by the right flank, he will command:

1. *Company, right*—FACE. 2. *Forward.* 3. MARCH.

136. At the first command, the company will face to the right, the covering sergeant will place himself at the head of the front rank, the captain having stepped out for the purpose, so far as to find himself by the side of the sergeant, and on his left: the front rank will double as is prescribed in the school of the soldier, No. 283; the rear rank will, at the same time, side step to the right one pace, and double in the same manner; so that when the movement is completed, the files will be formed of four men aligned, and elbow to elbow. The intervals will be preserved.

137. The file closers will also move by side step to the right, so that when the ranks are formed, they will be two paces from the rearmost rank.

138. At the command *march*, the company will move off brisk-ly in quick time; the covering sergeant at the head of the front rank, and the captain on his left, will march straight forward. The men of each file will march abreast of their respective front rank men, heads direct to the front: the file closers will march opposite their places in line of battle.

139. The instructor will cause the principles of the march by the flank to be observed, in placing himself, pending the march, as prescribed in the school of the soldier, No. 288.

140. The instructor will cause the march by the left flank to be executed by the same commands, substituting *left* for *right*; the ranks will double as has been prescribed in the school for the soldier, No. 285; the rear rank will side-step to the left one pace before doubling.

141. At the instant the company faces to the left, the left guide will place himself at the head of the front rank; the captain will pass rapidly to the left, and place himself by the right side of this guide; the covering sergeant will replace the captain in the front rank, the moment the latter quits it to go to the left.

ARTICLE SECOND.

*To change direction by file.*

142. The company being faced by the flank, and either in march, or at a halt, when the instructor shall wish to cause it to wheel by file, he will command:

1. *By file, left,* (or *right.*) 2. MARCH.

143. At the command *march*, the first file will wheel; if to the side of the front rank man, the latter will take care not to turn at

once, but to describe a short arc of a circle, shortening a little the first five or six steps in order to give time to the fourth man of this file to conform himself to the movement. If the wheel be to the side of the rear rank, the front rank man will wheel in the step of twenty-eight inches, and the fourth man will conform him. self to the movement by describing a short arc of a circle as has been explained. Each file will come to wheel on the same ground where that which preceded it wheeled.

144. The instructor will see that the wheel be executed according to these principles, in order that the distance between the files may always be preserved, and that there be no check or hindrance at the wheeling point.

### Article Third.

*To halt the company marching by the flank, and to face it to the front.*

145. To effect these objects, the instructor will command—

1. Company.   2. Halt.   3. Front.

146. The second and third commands will be executed as pre' scribed in the school of the soldier, Nos. 290 and 291. As soon as the files have undoubled, the rear rank will close to its proper distance. The captain and covering sergeant, as well as the left guide, if the march be by the left flank, will return to their habitual places in line at the instant the company faces to the front.

147. The instructor may then align the company, by one of the means prescribed, No. 100.

### Article Fourth.

*The company being in march by the flank, to form it on the right (or left) by file into line of battle.*

148. If the company be marching by the right flank, the instructor will command:

1. On the right, by file into line.   2. March.

149. At the command *march*, the rear rank men doubled will mark time; the captain and the covering sergeant will turn to the right, march straight forward, and be halted by the instructor when they shall have passed at least six paces beyond the rank of file closers; the captain will place himself correctly on the

line of battle, and will direct the alignment as the men of the front rank successively arrive ; the covering sergeant will place himself behind the captain at the distance of the rear rank ; the two men on the right of the front rank doubled, will continue to march, and passing beyond the covering sergeant and the captain, will turn to the right ; after turning, they will continue to march elbow to elbow, and direct themselves towards the line of battle, but when they shall arrive at two paces from this line, the even number will shorten the step so that the odd number may precede him on the line, the odd number placing himself by the side and on the left of the captain ; the even number will afterwards oblique to the left, and place himself on the left of the odd number; the next two men of the front rank doubled, will pass in the same manner behind the two first, turn then to the right, and place themselves, according to the means just explained, to the left, and by the side of, the two men already established on the line ; the remaining files of this rank will follow in succession, and be formed to the left in the same manner.  The rear rank doubled will execute the movement in the manner already explained for the front rank, taking care not to commence the movement until four men of the front rank are established on the line of battle ; the rear rank men, as they arrive on the line, will cover accurately their file leaders.

150. If the company be marching by the left flank, the instructor will cause it to form by file on the left into line of battle, according to the same principles and by the same commands, substituting the indication *left* for *right*.  In this case, the odd numbers will shorten the step, so that the even numbers may precede them on the line.  The captain, placed on the left of the front rank, and the left guide, will return to their places in line of battle, by order of the instructor, after the company shall be formed and aligned.

151. To enable the men the better to comprehend the mechanism of this movement, the instructor will at first cause it to be executed separately by each rank doubled, and afterwards by the two ranks united and doubled.

152. The instructor will place himself on the line of battle, and without the point where the right or left is to rest, in order to establish the base of the alignment, and afterwards, he will follow up the movement to assure himself that each file conforms itself to what is prescribed No. 149.

### ARTICLE FIFTH.

*The company being in march by the flank, to form it by company, or by platoon, into line, and to cause it to face to the right and left in marching.*

153. The company being in march by the right flank, the in-

structor will order the captain to form it into line ; the captain will immediately command :

1. *By company, into line* ; 2. MARCH.

154. At the command *march*, the covering sergeant will con. tinue to march straight forward; the men will advance the right shoulder, take the double quick step, and move into line, by the shortest route, taking care to undouble the files, and to come on the line one after the other.

155. As the front rank men successively arrive in line with the covering sergeant, they will take from him the step, and then turn their eyes to the front.

156. The men of the rear rank will conform to the movements of their respective file leaders, but without endeavoring to arrive in line at the same time with the latter.

157. At the instant the movement begins, the captain will face to his company in order to follow up the execution ; and, as soon as the company is formed, he will command, *guide left*, place himself two paces before the centre, face to the front, and take the step of the company.

158. At the command *guide left*, the second sergeant will promptly place himself in the front rank, on the left, to serve as guide, and the covering sergeant who is on the opposite flank will remain there.

159. When the company marches by the left flank, this move- ment will be executed by the same commands, and according to the same principles; the company being formed, the captain will command *guide right*, and place himself in front of his company as above ; the covering sergeant who is on the right of the front rank will serve as guide, and the second sergeant placed on the left flank will remain there.

160. Thus, in a column by company, right or left in front, the covering sergeant and the second sergeant of each company will always be placed on the right and left, respectively, of the front rank ; they will be denominated *right guide* and *left guide*, and the one or the other charged with the direction.

161. The company being in march by the flank, if it be the wish of the instructor to cause it to form platoons, he will give an order to that effect to the captain, who will command :

1. *By platoon, into line.* 2. MARCH.

162. The movement will be executed by each platoon accord- ing to the above principles. The captain will place himself be- fore the centre of the first platoon, and the first lieutenant before the centre of the second, passing through the opening made in the centre of the company, if the march be by the right flank, and around the left of his platoon, if the march be by the left : in this last

case, the captain will also pass around the left of the second platoon in order to place himself in front of the first. Both the captain and lieutenant, without waiting for each other, will command *guide left* (or *right*) at the instant their respective platoons are formed.

163. At the command *guide left* (or *right*,) the guide of each platoon will pass rapidly to the indicated flank of the platoon, if not already there.

164. The right guide of the company will always serve as the guide of the right or left of the first platoon, and the left guide of the company will serve, in like manner, as the guide of the second platoon.

165. Thus in a column, by platoon, there will be but one guide to each platoon; he will always be placed on its left flank, if the right be in front, and on the right flank, if the left be in front.

166. In these movements, the file closers will follow the platoons to which they are attached.

167. The instructor may cause the company, marching by the flank, to form by company, or by platoon, into line, by his own direct commands, using those prescribed for the captain, No. 153 or 161.

168. The instructor will exercise the company in passing, without a halt, from the march by the front, to the march by the flank, and reciprocally. In either case he will employ the commands prescribed in the school of the soldier, No. 294, substituting *company* for *squad*. The company will face to the right or left, in marching, and the captain, the guides, and file closers will conform themselves to what is prescribed for each in the march by the flank, or in the march by the front of a company supposed to be a subdivision of a column.

169. If, after facing to the right or left, in marching, the company find itself faced by the rear rank, the captain will place himself two paces behind the centre of the front rank, now in the rear, the guides will pass to the rear rank, now leading, and the file closers will march in front of this rank.

170. The instructor, in order to avoid fatiguing the men, and to prevent them from being negligent in the position of shoulder arms, will sometimes order support arms in marching by the flank, and arms on the right shoulder, when marching in line.

## LESSON FIFTH.

### ARTICLE FIRST.

*To break into column by platoon, either at a halt or in march.*

171. The company being at a halt, in line of battle, the instructor, wishing to break it into column, by platoon to the right, will command—

1. *By platoon, right wheel.*   2. MARCH.

172. At the first command, the chiefs of platoon will rapidly place themselves two paces before the centres of their respective platoons, the lieutenant passing around the left of the company. They need not occupy themselves with dressing, one upon the other. The covering sergeant will replace the captain in the front rank.

173. At the command *march*, the right front rank man of each platoon will face to the right, the covering sergeant standing fast; the chief of each platoon will move quickly by the shortest line, a little beyond the point at which the marching flank will rest when the wheel shall be completed, face to the late rear, and place himself so that the line which he forms with the man on the right (who had faced,) shall be perpendicular to that occupied by the company in line of battle ; each platoon will wheel according to the principles prescribed for the wheel on a fixed pivot, and when the man who conducts the marching flank shall approach near to the perpendicular, its chief will command :

1. *Platoon.*   2. HALT.

174. At the command *halt*, which will be given at the instant the man who conducts the marching flank shall have arrived at three paces from the perpendicular, the platoon will halt; the covering sergeant will move to the point where the left of the first platoon is to rest, passing by the front rank ; the second sergeant will place himself, in like manner, in respect to the second platoon. Each will take care to leave between himself and the man on the right of his platoon, a space equal to its front ; the captain and first lieutenant will look to this, and each take care to align the sergeant between himself and the man of the platoon who had faced to the right.

175. The guide of each platoon, being thus established on the perpendicular, each chief will place himself two paces outside of his guide, and facing towards him, will command :

3. *Left*—DRESS.

176. The alignment being ended, each chief of platoon will command, FRONT, and place himself two paces before its centre.

177. The file closers will conform themselves to the movement of their respective platoons, preserving always the distance of two paces from the rear rank.

178. The company will break by platoon to the left, according to the same principles. The instructor will command:

1. *By platoon, left wheel.*   2. MARCH.

179. The first command will be executed in the same manner as if breaking by platoon to the right.

180. At the command *march*, the left front rank man of each platoon will face to the left, and the platoons will wheel to the left, according to the principles prescribed for the wheel on a fixed pivot; the chiefs of platoon will conform to the principles indicated Nos. 173 and 174.

181. At the command *halt*, given by the chief of each platoon, the covering sergeant on the right of the front rank of the first platoon, and the second sergeant near the left of the second platoon, will each move to the points where the right of his platoon is to rest. The chief of each platoon should be careful to align the sergeant between himself and the man of the platoon who had faced to the left, and will then command:

### Right—Dress.

182. The platoons being aligned, each chief of platoon will command, Front, and place himself opposite its centre.

183. The instructor wishing to break the company by platoon to the right, and to move the column forward after the wheel is completed, will caution the company to that effect, and command:

### 1. *By platoon, right wheel.* 2. March.

184. At the first command, the chiefs of platoon will move rapidly in front of their respective platoons, conforming to what has been prescribed No. 172, and will remain in this position during the continuance of the wheel. The covering sergeant will replace the chief of the first platoon in the front rank.

185. At the command *march*, the platoons will wheel to the right, conforming to the principles herein prescribed; the man on the pivot will not face to the right, but will mark time, conforming himself to the movement of the marching flank; and when the man who is on the left of this flank shall arrive near the perpendicular, the instructor will command:

### 3. *Forward.* 4. March. 5. *Guide left.*

186. At the fourth command, which will be given at the instant the wheel is completed, the platoons will move straight to the front, all the men taking the step of twenty-eight inches. The covering sergeant and the second sergeant will move rapidly to the left of their respective platoons, the former passing before the front rank. The leading guide will immediately take points on the ground in the direction which may be indicated to him by the instructor.

187. At the fifth command, the men will take the touch of elbows lightly to the left.

188. If the guide of the second platoon should lose his distance, or the line of direction, he will conform to the principles herein prescribed Nos. 202 and 203.

189. If the company be marching in line to the front, the instructor will cause it to break by platoon to the right by the same commands. At the command *march*, the platoons will wheel in the manner already explained; the man on the pivot will take care to mark time in his place, without advancing or receding; the instructor, the chiefs of platoon, and the guides, will conform to what has been prescribed Nos. 184 and following.

190. The company may be broken by platoons to the left, according to the same principles, and by inverse means, the instructor giving the commands prescribed Nos. 183 and 185, substituting *left* for *right*, and reciprocally.

191. The movements explained in Nos. 183 and 189 will only be executed after the company has become well established in the principles of the march in column, Articles Second and Third.

### *Remarks.*

192. The instructor, placed in front of the company, will observe whether the movement be executed according to the principles prescribed above; whether the platoons, after breaking into column, are perpendicular to the line of battle just occupied; and whether the guide, who placed himself where the marching flank of his platoon had to rest, has left, between himself and the front rank man on the right (or left,) the space necessary to contain the front of the platoon.

193. After the platoons have broken, if the rearmost guide should not accurately cover the leading one, he will not seek to correct his position till the column be put in march, unless the instructor, wishing to wheel immediately into line, should think it necessary to rectify the direction of the guides, which would be executed as will be hereinafter explained in Article Fifth of this Lesson.

194. The instructor will observe, that the man on the right (or left) of each platoon, who, at the command *march*, faces to the right (or left) being the true pivot of the wheel, the front rank man next to him ought to gain a little ground to the front in wheeling, so as to clear the pivot-man.

### ARTICLE SECOND.

#### *To march in column.*

195. The company having broken by platoon, right (or left) in front, the instructor, wishing to cause the column to march, will throw himself twenty five or thirty paces in front, face to the

guides, place himself correctly, on their direction, and caution the leading guide to take points on the ground.

196. The instructor being thus placed, the guide of the leading platoon will take two points on the ground in the straight line passing between his own and the heels of the instructor.

197. These dispositions being made, the instructor will step aside, and command:

1. *Column, forward.*  2. *Guide left* (or *right.*)  3. MARCH.

198. At the command *march,* promptly repeated by the chiefs of platoon, they, as well as the guides, will lead off, by a decided step, their respective platoons, in order that the whole may move smartly, and at the same moment.

199. The men will each feel lightly the elbow of his neighbor towards the guide, and conform himself, in marching, to the principles prescribed in the school of the soldier, No. 253. The man next to the guide, in each platoon, will take care never to pass him, and also to march always about six inches to the right (or left) from him, in order not to push him out of the direction.

200. The leading guide will observe, with the greatest precision, the length and cadence of the step, and maintain the direction of his march by the means prescribed No. 89.

201. The following guide will march exactly in the trace of the leading one, preserving between the latter and himself a distance precisely equal to the front of his platoon, and marching in the same step with the leading guide.

202. If the following guide lose his distance from the one leading, (which can only happen by his own fault,) he will correct himself by slightly lengthening or shortening a few steps, in order that there may not be sudden quickenings or slackenings in the march of his platoon.

203. If the same guide, having neglected to march exactly in the trace of the preceding one, find himself sensibly out of the direction, he will remedy this fault by advancing more or less the shoulder opposite to the true direction, and thus, in a few steps, insensibly regain it, without the inconvenience of the oblique step, which would cause a loss of distance. In all cases, each chief of platoon will cause it to conform to the movements of its guide.

*Remarks on the march in column.*

204. If the chiefs and guides of subdivisions neglect to lead off and to decide the march from the first step, the march will be begun in uncertainty, which will cause waverings, a loss of step, and a loss of distance.

205. If the leading guide take unequal steps, the march of his subdivision, and that which follows, will be uncertain; there will be undulations, quickenings, and slackenings in the march.

206. If the same guide be not habituated to prolong a given direction, without deviation, he will describe a crooked line, and the column must wind to conform itself to such line.

207. If the following guide be not habituated to march in the trace of the preceding one, he will lose his distance at every moment in endeavors to regain the trace, the preservation of which is the most important principle in the march in column.

208. The guide of each subdivision in column will be responsible for the direction, distance and step; the chief of the subdivision, for the order and conformity of his subdivision with the movements of the guide. Accordingly, the chief will frequently turn, in the march, to observe his subdivision.

209. The instructor, placed on the flank of the guides, will watch over the execution of all the principles prescribed; he will, also, sometimes place himself in the rear, align himself on the guides, and halt, pending some thirty paces together, to verify the accuracy of the guides.

210. In column, chiefs of subdivision will always repeat, with the greatest promptitude, the commands *march* and *halt*, no chief waiting for another, but each repeating the command the moment he catches it from the instructor. They will repeat no other command given by him; but will explain, if necessary, to their subdivisions, in an under tone of voice, what they will have to execute, as indicated by the commands of caution.

### ARTICLE THIRD.
#### *To change direction.*

211. The changes of direction of a column while marching, will be executed according to the principles prescribed for wheeling on the march. Whenever, therefore, a column is to change direction, the instructor will change the guide, if not already there, to the flank opposite the side to which the change is to be made.

212. The column being in march right in front, if it be the wish of the instructor to change direction to the right, he will give the order to the chief of the first platoon, and immediately go himself, or send a marker to the point at which the change of direction is to be made; the instructor or marker, will place himself on the direction of the guides, so as to present the breast to that flank of the column.

213. The leading guide will direct his march on that person so that, in passing, his left arm may just graze his breast. When the leading guide shall have approached near to the marker, the chief of his platoon will command:

#### 1. *Right wheel.* 2. MARCH.

214. The first command will be given when the platoon is at the distance of four paces from the marker.

215. At the command *march,* which will be pronounced at the instant the guide shall have arrived opposite the marker, the platoon will wheel to the right, conforming to what is prescribed in the school of the soldier, No. 227.

216. The wheel being finished, the chief of each platoon will command:

3. *Forward.* 4. MARCH.

217. These commands will be pronounced and executed as prescribed in the school of the soldier, Nos. 229 and 230. The guide of the first platoon will take points on the ground in the new direction, in order the better to regulate the march.

218. The second platoon will continue to march straight forward till up with the marker, when it will wheel to the right, and retake the direct march by the same commands and the same means which governed the first platoon.

219. The column being in march right in front, if the instructor should wish to change the direction to the left, he will command, *guide right.* At this command, the two guides will move rapidly to the right of their respective platoons, each passing in front of his subdivision; the men will take the touch of elbows to the right; the instructor will afterwards conform to what is prescribed No. 212.

220. The change of direction to the left will then be executed acording to the same principles as the change of direction to the right, but by inverse means.

221. When the change of direction is completed, the instructor will command, *guide left.*

222. The changes of direction in a column, left in front, will be executed according to the same principles

223. In changes of direction in double quick time, the platoons will wheel according to the principles prescribed in the school of the soldier, No. 335.

224. In order to prepare the men for those formations in line, which can be executed only by turning to the right or the left, the instructor will sometimes cause the column to change direction to the side of the guide. In this case, the chief of the leading platoon will command: *Left* (or *right*) *turn,* instead of *left* or *right wheel.* The subdivisions will each turn, in succession, confirming to what is prescribed in the school of the soldier No. 333. The leading guide as soon as he has turned, will take points on the ground, the better to regulate the direction of the march.

225. It is highly important, in order to preserve distances and direction, that all the subdivisions of the column should change direction precisely at the point where the leading subdivision changed; it is for this reason that that point ought to be marked in advance, and that it is prescribed that the guides direct their march on the marker, also that each chief of subdivision shall

not cause the change to commence till the guide of his subdivision has grazed the breast of this marker.

226. Each chief will take care that his subdivision arrives at the point of change in a square with the line of direction : with this view, he will face to his subdivision when the one which precedes has commenced to turn or to wheel, and he will be watchful that it continues to march squarely until it arrives at the point where the change of direction is to commence.

227. If, in changes of direction, the pivot of the subdivision which wheels should not clear the wheeling point, the next subdivision would be arrested and distances lost ; for the guide who conducts the marching flank having to describe an arc, in length about a half greater than the front of the subdivision, the second subdivision would be already up with the wheeling point, whilst the first which wheels has yet the half of its front to execute, and hence would be obliged to mark time until that half be executed. It is therefore prescribed, that the pivot of each subdivision should take steps of nine or eleven inches in length, according the the swiftness of the gait, in order not to arrest the march of the next subdivision. The chiefs of subdivision will look well to the step ot the pivot, and cause his step to be lengthened or shortened as may be judged necessary. By the nature of this movement, the centre of each subdivision will bend a little to the rear.

221. The guides will never alter the length or cadence of the step, whether the change of direction be to the side of the guide or to the opposite side.

229. The marker, placed at the wheeling point, will always present his breast to the flank of the column. The instructor will take the greatest pains in causing the prescribed principles to be observed ; he will see that each subdivision only commences the change of direction when the guide, grazing the breast of the marker, has nearly passed him, and, that the marching flank does not describe the arc ot too large a circle, in order that it may not be thrown beyond the new direction.

230. In change of direction by wheel, the guide of the wheeling flank will cast his eyes over the ground at the moment of commencing the wheel, and will describe an arc of a circle whose radius is equal to the front of the subdivision.

### Article Fourth.

*To halt the column.*

231. The column being in march, when the instructor shall wish to halt it, he will command :

1. *Column.*   2. Halt.

232. At the second command, promptly repeated by the chiefs of platoon, the column will halt ; the guides also will stand fast, although they may have lost both distance and direction.

233. If the command *halt*, be not repeated with the greatest vivacity, and executed at the same instant, distances will be lost.

234. If a guide, having lost his distance, seek to recover it after that command, he will only throw his fault on the following guide, who, if he have marched well, will no longer be at his proper distance ; and if the latter regain what he has thus lost, the movement will be propagated to the rear of the column.

### ARTICLE FIFTH.

*Being in column by platoon, to form to the right or left into line of battle, either at a halt or on the march.*

235. The instructor having halted the column, right in front, and wishing to form it into line of battle, will place himself at platoon distance in front of the leading guide, face to him, and rectify, if necessary, the position of the guide beyond : which being executed, he will command :

### *Left*—DRESS.

236. At this command, which will not be repeated by the chiefs of platoon, each of them will place himself briskly two paces outside of his guide, and direct the alignment of the platoon perpendicularly to the direction of the column.

237. Each chief having aligned his platoon, will command FRONT, and return quickly to his place in column.

238. This disposition being made, the instructor will command :

1. *Left into line, wheel.*  2. MARCH.

239. At the command *march*, briskly repeated by the chiefs of platoon, the front rank men on the left of each platoon will face to the left, and place his breast lightly against the arm of the guide by his side, who stands fast ; the platoons will wheel to the left on the principle of wheels from a halt, and in conformity to what is prescribed 125. Each chief will turn to his platoon to observe its movement, and when the marching flank has approached near the line of battle, he will command :

1. *Platoon.*  2. HALT.

240. The command *halt* will be given when the marching

flank of the platoon is three paces from the line of battle.

241. The chief of the second platoon, having halted it, will return to his place as a file closer, passing around the left of his subdivision.

242. The captain having halted the first platoon, will move rapidly to the point at which the right of the company will rest in line of battle, and command :

*Right*—Dress.

243. At this command, the two platoons will dress up on the alignment ; the front rank man on the right of the leading platoon, who finds himself opposite the instructor established on the direction of the guides, will place his breast lightly against the left arm of this officer. The captain will direct the alignment from the right on the man on the opposite flank of the company.

244. The company being aligned, the captain will command:

Front.

245. The instructor seeing the company in line of battle, will command :

*Guides*—Posts.

1. *Right into line wheel.*  2. March.

246. At this command, the covering sergeant will cover the captain, and the left guide will return to his place as a file closer.

247. If the column be left in front, and the instructor should wish to form it to the right into line of battle, he will place himself at platoon distance in front of the leading guide, face to him, and rectify, if necessary, the position of the guide beyond ; which being executed, he will command :

248. At the command *march*, the front rank man on the right of each platoon will face to the right and place his breast lightly against the left arm of the guide by his side, who stands fast; each platoon will wheel to the right, and will be halted by its chief, when the marching flank has approached near the line of battle ; for this purpose, the chief of each platoon will command :

1. *Platoon.*  2. Halt.

249. The command *halt*, will be given when the marching flank of the platoon is three paces from the line of battle.

The chief of the second platoon having halted his platoon, will resume his place in the rank of file closers.

250. The captain having halted the first platoon, will move briskly to the point at which the left of the company will rest, and command :

*Left*—DRESS.

251. At this command, the two platoons will dress up on the alignment ; the man on the left of the second platoon, opposite the instructor, will place his breast lightly against the right arm of his officer, and the captain will direct the alignment from the left on the man on the opposite flank of the company.

252. The company being aligned, the captain will command :

FRONT.

253. The instructor will afterwards command :

*Guides*—POSTS.

254. At this command, the captain will move to the right of his company; the covering sergeant will cover him, and the left guide will return to his place as a file closer.

255. The instructor may omit the command *left* or *right dress*, previous to commanding *left* or *right into line, wheel*, unless, after rectifying the position of the guides, it should become necessary to redress the platoons, or one of them, latterally to the right or left.

256. The instructor, before the command *left (or right) into line, wheel*, will assure himself that the rearmost platoon is at its exact wheeling distance from the one in front. This attention is important, in order to detect negligence on the part of guides in this essential point.

257. If the column be marching right in front, and the instructor should wish to form it into line without halting the column, he will give the command prescribed No. 169, and move rapidly to platoon distance in front of the leading guide.

258. At the command *march*, briskly repeated by the chiefs the left guides will halt short, the instructor, the chiefs of platoon, and the p'atoons, will conform to what is prescribed No. 160 and following.

259. If the column be in march left in front, this formation will be made according to the same principles, and by inverse means.

260. If the column be marching right in front, and the instructor should wish to form it into line without halting the column, and to march the company in line to the front, he will command :

1. *By platoons left wheel* 2. MARCH.

261. At the command *march*, briskly repeated by the chiefs of platoon, the left guides will halt: the man next to the left guide in each platoon will mark time : the platoons will wheel to the left, conforming to the principles of the wheel on a fixed pivot. When the right of the platoons shall arrive near the line of battle, the instructor will command :

3. *Forward.* 4. MARCH. 5. *Guide right (or left.)*

262. At the fourth command, given at the instance the wheel is completed, all the men of the company will move off together with the step of twenty-eight inches ; the captain, the chief of the second platoon, the covering sergeant, and the left guide will take their position as in line of battle.

263. At the fifth command, which will be given immediately after the fourth, the captain and covering sergeant, if not already there, will move briskly to the side on which the guide is designated. The non-commissioned officer charged with the direction will move rapidly in front of the guide, and will be assured in his line of march by the instructor, as is prescribe t No. 104'. That non-commissioned officer will immediately take points on the ground as indicated in the same number. The men will take the touch of elbows to the side of the guide, conforming themselves to the principle of the march in line.

264. The same principles are applicable to a column left in front.

## LESSON SIXTH.

### ARTICLE FIRST.

*To break the company into platoons, and to re-form the company.*

*To break the company into platoons.*

265. The company marching in the cadenced step, and supposed to make part of a column, right in front, when the instructor shall wish to cause it to break by platoons, he will give the order to the captain, who will command: 1. *Break into platoons,* and immediately place himself before the centre of the first platoon.

266. At the command *break into platoons,* the first lieutenant will pass quickly around the left, to the centre of his platoon, and give the caution : *Mark time.*

267. The captain will then command : 2. *March.*

268. The first platoon will continue to march straight forward ; the covering sergeant will move rapidly to the left flank of this platoon (passing by the front rank) as soon as the flank shall be disengaged.

269. At the command *march*, given by the captain, the second platoon will begin to matk time ; its chief will immediately add : 1. *Right oblique ;* 2. MARCH. The last command will be given so that this platoon may commence obliquing the instant the rear rank of the first platoon shall have passed. The men will shorten the step in obliquing, so that when the command *forward march* is given, the platoon may have its exact distance.

270. The guide of the second platoon being near the direction of the guide of the first, the chief of the second will command *Forward*, and add MARCH, the instant that the guide of his platoon shall cover the guide of the first.

271. In a column, left in front, the company will break into platoons by inverse means, applying to the first platoon all that has been prescribed for the second, and reciprocally.

272. In this case, the left guide of the company will shift to the right flank of the second platoon, and the covering sergeant will remain on the right of the first.

*To re-form the company.*

273 The column, by platoon, being in march, right in front, when the instructor shall wish to cause it to form company, he will give the order to the captain, who will command : *Form company.*

274. Having given this command, the captain will immediately add : 1. *First Platoon ;* 2. *Right oblique.*

275. The chief of the second platoon will caution it to continue to march straight forward.

276. The captain will then command : 3. MARCH.

277. At this command, repeated by the chief of the second, the first platoon will oblique to the right, in order to unmask the second ; the covering sergeant, on the left of the first platoon, will return to the right of the company, passing by the front rank.

278. When the first platoon shall have nearly unmasked the second, the captain will command : 1. *Mark time,* and at the instant the unmasking shall be complete; he will add : 2. MARCH. The first platoon will then cease to oblique, and mark time.

280. In the mean time the second platoon will have continued to march straight forward, and when it shall be nearly up with the first, the captain will command *Forward,* and at the instant the two platoons shall unite, add MARCH ; the first platoon will then cease to mark time.

280. In a column, left in front the same movement will be executed by inverse means, the chief of the second platoon giving the command *Forward,* and the captain adding the command MARCH, when the platoons are united.

281. The guide of the second platoon, on its right, will pass

to its left flank the moment the platoon begins to oblique ; the
guide of the first, on its right, rema ning on that flank of the
platoon.

282. The instructor will also sometimes cause the company to
break and re-form, by platoon, by his own direct commands.—
In this case, he will give the general commands prescribed for
the captain above : 1. *Break into platoons ;* 2. MARCH ; and 1.
*Form company* ; 2 MARCH.

283. If, in breaking the company into platoons, the subdivision that breaks off should mark time too long, it might, in a
column of many subdivisions, arrest the march of the following one, which would cause a lengthening of the column, and a
loss of distances.

284. In breaking into platoons, it is necessary that the platoons
which oblique should not shorten the step too much, in order not
to lose distance in column, and not to arrest the march of the
following subdivision.

275. If a platoon obliques too far to a flank, it would be
obliged to oblique again to the opposite flank, to regain the direction, and by the double movement arrest probably, the march
of the following subdivision.

286. The chiefs of those platoons which oblique will face
to their platoons, in order to enforce the observance of the fore-
going principles.

287. When, in a column of several companies, they break in
succession, it is of the greatest importance that each company
should continue to march in the same st p, without shortening
or slackening, whilst that which precedes breaks, although the
following company should close up on the preceding one. This
attention is essential to guard against an elongation of the
column.

288. Faults of but little moment, in a column of a few companies, would be serious inconveniences in a general column
of many battalions. Hence the instructor will give the greatest
care in causing all the prescribed principles to be strictly observed. To this end, he will hold himself on the directing
flank, the better to observe all the movements

## ARTICLE SECOND.

*Being in column, to break files to the rear, and to cause them to
re-enter into line.*

289. The company being in march, and supposed to constitute
a subdivision of a column, right (or left) in front, when the
instructor shall wish to cause files to break off he will give the
order to the captain, who will immediately turn to his company,
d command :

1. *Two files from left* (or *right*) *to rear.* 2. MARCH.

290. At the command *march*, the two files on the left (or right) of the company will mark time, the others will continue to march straight forward ; the two rear rank men of these files will, as soon as the rear rank of the company shall clear them. move to the right by advancing the outer shoulder ; the odd number will place himself behind the third file from that flank, the even number behind the fourth, passing for this purpose behind the odd number ; the two front rank men will, in like manner, move to the right when the rear rank of the company shall clear them, the odd number will place himself behind the first file, the even number behind the second file, passing for this purpose behind the odd number. If the files are broken from the right, the men will move to the left, advancing the outer shoulder, the even number of the rear rank will place himself behind the third file, the odd number of the same rank behind the fourth ; the even number of the front rank behind the first file, the odd number of the same rank behind the second, the odd numbers for this purpose passing the even numbers. The men will be careful not to lose their distances and to keep aligned.

291. If the instructor should wish to break two files from the same side, he will give the order to the captain, who will proceed as above directed.

292. At the command *march*, given by the captain, the files already broken, advancing a little the outer shoulder, will gain the space of two files to the right, if the files are broken from the left, and to the left, if the files are broken from the right. shortening, at the same time, the step, in order to make room between themselves and the rear rank of the company for the files last ordered to the rear ; the latter will break by the same commands and in the same manner as the first. The men who double should increase the length of the step in order to prevent distances from being lost.

293. The instructor may thus diminish the front of a company by breaking off successive groups of two files, but the new files must always be broken from the same side.

294. The instructor, wishing to cause the files broken off to return into line, will give the order to the captain, who will immediately command :

1. *Two files into line.* 2. MARCH.

295. At the command *march*, the first two files of those marching by the flank will return briskly into line, and the others will gain the space of two files by advancing the inner shoulder towards the flank to which they belong.

296. The captain will turn to his company to watch the observance of the principles which have just been prescribed.

297. The instructor having caused groups of two files to

break one after another, and to return again into line, will afterwards cause two or three groups to break together, and for this purpose will command : *Four or six files from left* (or *right*) *to the rear ;* MARCH. The files designated will mark time ; each rank will advance a little the outer shoulder as soon as the rear rank of the company shall clear it, will oblique at once, and each group will place itself behind the four neighboring files, and in the same manner, as if the movement had been executed group by group, taking care that the distances are preserved.

298. The instructor will next order the captain to cause two or three groups to be brought into line at once, who, turning to the company, will command :

*Four or six files into line—*MARCH.

299. At the command *march*, the files designated will advance the inner shoulder, move up and form on the flank of the company by the shortest lines.

300. As often as files shall break off to the rear, the guide on that flank will gradually close on the nearest front rank man remaining in line, and he will also open out to make room for files ordered into line.

301. The files which march in the rear are disposed in the following order : the left files as if the company was marching by the right flank, and the right files as if the company were marching by the left flank. Consequently, whenever there is on the right or left of a subdivision, a file which does not belong to a group, it will be broken singly.

302. It is necessary to the preservation of distances in column that the men should be habituated in the schools of detail to execute the movements of this article with precision.

303. If new files broken off do not step well to the left or right in obliquing ; if, when files are ordered into line, they do not move up with promptitude and precision, in either case the following files will be arrested in their march, and thereby cause the column to be lengthened out.

304. The instructor will place himself on the flank from which the files are broken, to assure himself of the exact observance of the principles.

305. Files will only be broken off from the side of direction, in order that the whole company may easily pass from the front to the flank march.

ARTICLE THIRD.

*To march the column in route, and to execute the movements incident thereto.*

306. The swiftness of the route step will be one hundred

and ten steps in a minute ; this swiftness will be habitually maintained in column in route, when the roads and ground may permit.

'307. The company being at a halt, and supposed to constitute a subdivision of a column, when the instructor shall wish to cause it to march in the route step, he will command :

1. *Column, forward.* 2. *Guide, left* (or *right.*) 3. *Route step.*
4. March.

308. At the command *march*, repeated by the captain, the two ranks will step off together ; the rear rank will take, in marching, by shortening a few steps, a distance of one pace, (twenty-eight inches) from the rank preceding, which distance will be computed from the breasts of the men in the rear rank, to the knapsacks of the men in the front rank. The men, without further command, will immediately carry their arms *at will*, as indicated in the school of the soldier, No. 140. They will no longer be required to march in the cadence pace, or with the same foot, or to remain silent. The files will march at ease ; but care will be taken to prevent the ranks from intermixing, the front rank from getting in advance of the guide, and the rear rank from opening to too great a distance.

309. The company marching in the route step, the instructor will cause it to change direction, which will be executed without formal commands, on a simple caution from the captain ; the rear rank will come up to change direction in the same manner as the front rank. Each rank will conform itself, although in the route step, to the principles which have been prescribed for the change in closed ranks, with this difference only : that the pivot man, instead of taking steps of nine, will take steps of fourteen inches, in order to clear the wheeling point.

310. The company marching in the route step, to cause it to pass to the cadenced step, the instructor will first order pieces to be brought to the right shoulder, and then command :

1. *Quick time.* 2. March.

311. At the command *march*, the men will resume the cadenced step, and will close so as to leave a distance of sixteen inches between each rank.

312. The company marching in the cadenced pace, the instructor, to cause it to take the route step, will command :

1. *Route step.* 2. March.

313. At the command *march*, the front rank will continue the step of twenty-eight inches, the rear rank will take, by

gradually shortening the step, the distance of twenty-eight inches from the front rank ; the men will carry their arms at will.

314. If the company be marching in the route step, and the instructor should suppose the necessity of marching by the flank in the same direction, he will command :

1. *Company by the right* (or *left*) *flank.*   2. *By file left* (or *right.*)   3. MARCH.

315. At the command *march*, the company will face to the right (or left) in marching, the captain will place himself by the side of the guide who conducts the leading flank ; this guide will wheel immediately to the left or right ; all the files will come in succession to wheel on the same spot as the guide ; if there be files broken off to the rear, they will, by wheeling, regain their respective places, and follow the movement of the company.

316. The instructor, having caused the company to be again formed into line, will exercise it in increasing and diminishing front, by platoon, which will be executed by the same commands, and the same means, as if the company were marching in the cadenced step. When the company breaks into platoons, the chief of each will move to the flank of his platoon, and will take the place of the guide, who will step back into the rear rank.

317. The company being in column, by platoon, and supposed to march in the route step, the instructor can cause the front to be diminished and increased, by section, if the platoons have a front of twelve files or more.

318. The movements of diminishing and increasing front, by section, will be executed according to the principles indicated for the same movement by platoons. The right sections of platoons will be commanded by the captain and first lieutenant, respectively ; the left sections, by the two next subalterans in rank, or, in their absence, by sergeants.

319. The instructor, wishing to diminish by section, will give the order to the captain, who will command :

1. *Break into sections.*   2. MARCH.

320. As soon as the platoons shall be broken, each chief of section will place himself on its directing flank in the front rank; the guides who will be thus displaced, will fall back into the rear rank; the file closer will close up to within one pace of this rank.

321. Platoons will be broken into sections only in the column in route, the movement will never be executed in the

manœuvres, whatever may be the front of the company.

322. When the instructor shall wish to re-form platoons, he will give the order to the captain, who will command:.

1. *Form platoons.*  2. March.

323. At the first command, each chief of section will place himself before its centre, and the guides will pass into the front rank. At the command *march*, the movement will be executed as has been prescribed for forming company. The moment the platoons are formed, the chiefs of the left sections will return to their places as file closers.

324. The instructor will also cause to be executed the diminishing and increasing front by files, as prescribed in the preceding article, and in the same manner, as if marching in the cadenced step. When the company is broken into sections, the subdivisions must not be reduced to a front of less than six files, not counting the chief of the section.

325. The company being broken by platoon, or by section, the instructor will cause it, marching in the route step, to march by the flank in the same direction, by the commands and the means indicated, Nos. 314 and 315. The moment the subdivisions shall face to the right (or left,) the first file of each will wheel to the left (or right,) in marching, to prolong the direction, and to unite with the rear file of the subdivision immediately preceding. The file closers will take their habitual places in the march by the flank, before the union of the subdivisions.

326. If the company be marching by the right flank, and the instructor should wish to undouble the files, which might sometimes be found necessary, he will inform the captain, who, after causing the cadenced step to be resumed, and arms to be shouldered or supported, will command :

1. *In two ranks, undouble file.*  2. March.

327. At the second command, the odd numbers will continue to march straight forward the even numbers will shorten the step, and obliquing to the left will place themselves promptly behind the odd numbers; the rear rank will gain a step to the left so as to re-take the touch of elbows on the side of the front rank

328 If the company be marching by the left flank, it will be the even numbers who will continue to march forward, and the odd numbers who will undouble.

329. If the instructor should wish to double the files, he will give the order to the captain, who will command:

1. *In four ranks, double files.*  2 March.

330. At the command *march*, the files will double in the manner as explained, when the company faces by the right or the left flank. The instructor will afterwards cause the route step to be resumed.

331. The various movements prescribed in this lesson may be executed in double quick time. The men will be brought, by degrees, to pass over at this gait about eleven hundred yards in seven minutes.

332 When the company marching in the route step shall halt, the rear rank will close up at the command *halt*, and the whole will shoulder arms.

333. Marching in the route step, the men will be permitted to carry their pieces in the manner they shall find most convenient, paying attention only to hold the muzzles up, so as to avoid accidents.

ARTICLE FOURTH.

*Countermarch.*

334. The company being at a halt, and supposed to constitute part of a column, right in front, when the instructor shall wish to cause it to countermarch, he will command :

1. *Countermarch.*   2. *Company, right*—FACE.   3. *By file left.*
4. MARCH.

335. At the second command, the company will face to the right, the two guides to the right about ; the captain will go to the right of his company and cause two files to break to the rear, and then place himself by the side of the front rank man, to conduct him.

336. At the command *march*, both guides will stand fast ; the company will step off smartly ; the first file, conducted by the captain, will wheel around the right guide, and direct its march along the front rank so as to arrive behind, and two paces from the left guide ; each file will come in succession to wheel on the same ground around the right guide ; the leading file having arrived at a point opposite to the left guide, the captain will command :

1. *Company.*   2. HALT.   3. FRONT.   4. *Right*—DRESS.

337. The first command will be given at *four* paces from the point where the leading file is to rest.

338. At the second command, the company will halt.

339. At the third, it will face to the front.

340. At the fourth, the company will dress by the right ; the captain will step two paces outside of the left guide, now on the right, and direct the alignment, so that the front rank may be enclosed between the two guides ; the company being

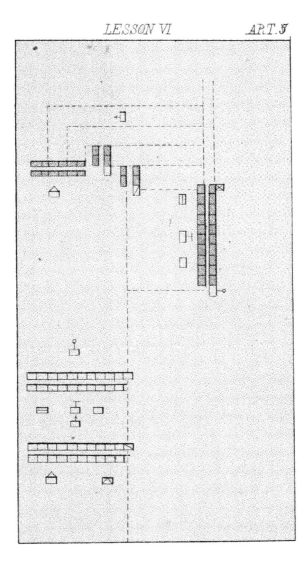

aligned, he will command FRONT, and place himself before the centre of the company as if in column ; the guides, passing along the front rank, will shift to their proper places, on the right and left of that rank.

341. In a column, by platoon, the countermarch will be executed by the same commands, and according to the same principles ; the guide of each platoon will face about, and its chief will place himself by the side of the file on the right, to conduct it.

342. In a column, left in front, the countermarch will be executed by inverse commands and means, but according to the same principles. Thus, the movement will be made by the right flank of subdivisions, if the right be in front, and by the left flank, if the left be in front ; in both cases the subdivisions will wheel by file to the side of the front rank.

### ARTICLE FIFTH.

*Being in column by platoon, to form on the right (or left) into line of battle.*

343. The column by platoon, right in front, being in march, the instructor, wishing to form it on the right into line of battle, will command :

1. *On the right into line.* 2. *Guide right.*

344. At the second command, the guide of each platoon will shift quickly to its right flank, and the men will touch elbows to the right ; the column will continue to march straight forward.

345. The instructor having given the second command, will move briskly to the point at which the right of the company ought to rest in line, and place himself facing the point of direction to the left which he will choose.

346. The line of battle ought to be so chosen that the guide of each platoon, after having turned to the right, may have, at least, ten paces to take before arriving upon that line.

347. The head of the column being nearly opposite to the instructor, the chief of the first platoon will command : 1. *Right turn ;* and when exactly opposite to that point, he will add :

2. MARCH.

348. At the command *march*, the first platoon will turn to the right, in conformity with the principles prescribed in the school of the soldier, No. 333. Its guide will so direct his march as to bring the front rank man, next on his left, oppo-

site to the instructor ; the chief of the platoon will march
before its centre ; and when its guide shall be near the line
of battle, he will command :

1 *Platoon.*    2. HALT.

349. At the command *halt*, which will be given at the instant the right of the platoon shall arrive at the distance of
three paces from the line of battle, the platoon will halt ;
the files, not yet in line, will come up promptly. The guide
will throw himself on the line of battle, opposite to one of
of the three left files of his platoon ; he will face to the instructor, who will align him on the point of direction to the
left. The chief of platoon having, at the same time gone to
the point where the right of the company is to rest, will, as
soon as he sees all the files of the platoon in line, command :

*Right*—DRESS.

350. At this the first platoon will align itself ; the front
rank man, who finds himself opposite to the guide, will rest
his breast lightly against the right arm of this guide, and
the chief of the platoon, from the right, will direct the alignment on this man.

351. The second platoon will continue to march straight
forward, until its guide shall arrive opposite to the left file
of the first ; it will then turn to the right at the command of
its chief, and march towards the line of battle, its guide directing himself on the left file of the first platoon.

352. The guide having arrived at the distance of three
paces from the line of battle, this platoon will be halted, as
prescribed for the first : at the instant it halts, its guide will
spring on the line of battle, opposite to one of the three left
files of his platoon, and will be assured in his position by the
instructor.

353. The chief of the second platoon, seeing all its files in
line, and its guide established on the direction, will command :

*Right* —DRESS

354. Having given this command, he will return to his
place as a file closer, passing around the left ; the second
platoon will dress up on the alignment of the first, and when
established, the captain will command :

FRONT.

355. The movement ended, the instructor will command :

*Guides*—POSTS

356. At this command, the two guides will return to their places in line of battle.

357. A column, by platoon, left in front, will form on the left into line of battle, according to the same principles, and, by inverse means, applying to the second platoon what is prescribed for the first, and reciprocally. The chief of the second platoon having aligned it, from the point of *appui*, (the left,) will retire to his place as a file closer. The captain having halted the first platoon three paces behind the line of battle, will go the same point to align this platoon, and then command : FRONT. At the command, *guides—posts*, given by the instructor, the captain will shift to his proper flank, and the guides take their places in the line of battle.

358. When the companies of a regiment are be exercised, at the same time, in the school of the company, the colonel will indicate the lesson or lessons they are severally to execute. The whole will commence by a bugle signal, and terminate in like manner.

*Formation of a company from two ranks into single rank, and reciprocally.*

359. The company being formed into two ranks in the manner indicated No 8, school of the soldier, and supposed to make part of a column, right or left in front, when the instructor shall wish to form into single rank, he will command :

1. *In one rank, form company.* 2. MARCH.

360. At the first command, the right guide will face to the right.

361. At the command *march*, the right guide will step off and march in the prolongation of the front rank.

362. The first file will step off at the same time with the guide ; the front rank man will turn to the right at the first step, follow the guide, and be himself followed by the rear rank man of his file, who will come to turn on the same spot where he had turned. The second file, and successively all the other files, will step off as has been prescribed for the first, the front rank man of each file following immediately the rear rank man of the file next on his right. The captain will superintend the movement, and when the last man shall have stepped off, he will halt the company, and face it to the front.

363. The file closers will take their places in line of battle, two paces in rear of the rank.

364. The company being in single rank, when the instructor shall wish to form it into two ranks, he will command :

1. *In two ranks, form company.*    2. *Company: right—*FACE.
3. MARCH.

365. At the second command, the company will face to the right : the right guide and the man on the right will remain faced to the front.

366. At the command *march;* the men who have faced to the right, will step off, and form files in the following manner : the second man in the rank will place himself behind the first to form the first file ; the third will place himself by the side of the first in the front rank ; the fourth behind the third in the rear rank. All the others will, in like manner, place themselves, alternately, in the front and rear rank, and will thus form files of two men, on the left of those already formed.

367. The formations above described will be habitually executed by the right of companies ; but when the instructo shall wish to have them executed by the left, he will face the company *about,* and post the guides in the rearrank.

368. The formation will then be executed by the same commands, and according to the same principles as by the front rank ; the movement commencing with the left file, now become the right, and in each file by the rear rank man, now become the front ; the left guide will conform to what has been prescribed for the right.

369. The formation ended, the instructor will face the company to its proper front.

370. When a battalion in line has to execute either of the formations above described, the colonel will cause it to break to the rear by the right or left of companies, and will then give the commands just prescribed for the instructor. Each company will execute the movement as if acting singly.

*Formation of a company from two ranks into four, and reciprocally, at a halt, and in march.*

371. The company being formed in two ranks, at a halt, and supposed to form a part of a column right in front, when the instructor shall wish to form it into four ranks, he will command :

1. *In four ranks, form company.*    2. *Company left—*FACE.
3. MARCH (or *double quick—*MARCH ).

372. At the second command, the left guide will remain faced to the front, the company will face to the left : the rear rank will gain the distance of one pace from the front

rank by a side step to the left and rear, and the men will form into four ranks as prescribed in the school of the soldier.

3.73. At the command *march*, the first file of four men will reface to the front without undoubling. All the other files of four will step off, and closing successively to about five inches of the preceding file, will halt, and immediately face to the front, the men remaining doubled.

374. The file closers will take their new places in line of battle, at two paces in rear of the fourth rank.

375. The captain will superintend the movement.

376. The company being in four ranks, when the instructor shall wish to form it into two ranks, he will command :

1. *In two ranks, form company.* 2. *Company right—*FACE. 3. MARCH (or *double quick—*MARCH.)

377. At the second command the left guide will stand fast, the company will face to the right.

378. At the command *march*, the right guide will step off, and march in the prolongation of the front rank. The leading file of four men will step off at the same time, the other files standing fast ; the second file will step off when there shall be between it and the first space sufficient to form into two ranks. The following files will execute successively what has been prescribed for the second. As soon as the last file shall have its distance, the instructor will command :

1. *Company.* 2. HALT. 3. FRONT.

379. At the command *front*, the company will face to the front, and the files will undouble.

380. The company being formed in two ranks, and marching to the front, when the instructor shall wish to form it into four ranks, he will command :

1. *In four ranks, form company.* 2. *By the left, double files.* 3. MARCH (or *double quick—*MARCH.)

381. At the command *march*, the left guide and the left file of the company will continue to march straight to the front : the company will make a half face to the left, the odd numbers placing themselves behind the even numbers. The even numbers of the rear rank will shorten their steps a little to permit the odd numbers of the front rank to get between them and the even numbers of that rank. The files thus formed of fours, except the left file, will continue to march obliquely, lengthening their steps slightly, so as to keep constantly abreast of the guide; each file will close suc-

cessively on the file next on its left, and when at the proper distance from that file, will face to the front by a half face to the right, and take the touch of elbows to the left.

382. The company being in march to the front in four ranks, when the instructor shall wish to form it in two ranks, he will command :

1. *In two ranks, form company.*   2. *By the right, undouble files.*
3. March (or *double quick*—March )

383. At the command *march*, the left guide and the left file of the company will continue to march straight to the front ; the company will make a half face to the right and march obliquely, lengthening the step a little, in order to keep, as near as possible, abreast of the guide.   As soon as the second file from the left shall have gained to the right the interval necessary for the left file to form into two ranks, the second file will face to the front by a half face to the left and march straight forward ; the left file will immediately form into two ranks, and take the touch of elbows to the left.   Each file will execute successively, what has just been prescribed for the file next to the left, and each file will form into two ranks when the file next on its right has obliqued the required distance and faced to the front.

384. If the company be supposed to make part of a column, left in front, these different movements will be executed according to the same principles and by inverse means, substituting the indication *left* for *right.*

END OF THE SCHOOL OF THE COMPANY.

# INSTRUCTIONS FOR SKIRMISHERS.

## *General Principles and Division of the Instruction.*

1. The movements of Skirmishers should be subjected to such rules as will give to the commander the means of moving them in any direction with the greatest promptitude,

2. It is not expected that these movements should be executed with the same precision as in closed ranks, nor is it desirable, as such exactness would interfere with their prompt execution.

3. When Skirmishers are thrown out to clear the way for, and to protect the advance of, the main corps, their movements must be so regulated by this corps, as to keep it constantly covered.

4. Every body of Skirmishers should have a reserve, the strength of which will vary according to circumstances.

5. If the body thrown out be within sustaining distance of the main corps, a small reserve will be sufficient for each company, whose duty it shall be to fill vacant places, furnish the line with cartridges, relieve the fatigued, and serve as rallying points.

6. If the main corps be at a considerable distance, besides the company reserves, another reserve will be required, composed of entire companies, which will sustain and reinforce such parts of the line as may be attacked; this reserve should be strong enough to relieve half the companies deployed as skirmishers.

7. The reserves should be placed behind the centre of the line of skirmishers, the company reserves at 150, and the principal reserve at 400 paces. This, rule, however, is not invariable.— The reserves, while holding themselves within sustaining distance of the line, should be, as much as possible, in position to afford each other mutual protection, and must carefully profit by any accidents of the ground to conceal themselves from the view of the enemy and to shelter themselves from his fire.

8. The movements of Skirmishers will be executed in quick, or double quick time. The run will be resorted to only in cases of urgent necessity.

9. Skirmishers will be permitted to carry their pieces in the manner most convenient to them.

10. The movements will be habitually indicated by the sounds of the bugle.

11. The officers and non-commissioned officers will repeat, and couse the commands to be executed, as soon as they

13

are given; but to avoid mistakes, when the signals are employed they will wait until the last bugle note is sounded before commencing the movement.

12. When skirmishers are ordered to move rapidly, the officers and non-commisioned officers will see that the men economise their strength, keep cool, and profit by all the advantages which the ground may offer for cover. It is only by this continual watchfulness on the part of all grades, that a line of skirmishers can attain success.

13. This instruction will be divided into five articles, and subdivided as follows:

### ARTICLE FIRST.

1. To deploy forward.
2. To deploy by the flank.
3. To extend intervals.
4. To close intervals.
5. To relieve skirmishers.

### ARTICLE SECOND.

1. To advance in line.
2. To retreat in line.
3. To change direction.
4. To march by the flank.

### ARTICLE THIRD.

1. To fire at a halt.
2. To fire marching.

### ARTICLE FOURTH.

1. The rally.
2. To form column to march in any direction.
3. The assembly.

### ARTICLE FIFTH.

1. To deploy a battalion as skirmishers.
2. To rally the battalion deployed as skirmishers.

14. In the first four articles, it is supposed that the movements are executed by a company deployed as skirmishers, on a front equal to that of the battalion in order of battle. In the fifth article, it is supposed that each company of the battalion, being deployed as skirmishers, occupies a front of one hundred paces. From these two examples, rules may be deduced for all cases, whatever may be the numerical strength of the skirmishers, and the extent of ground they ought to occupy.

### ARTICLE FIRST.

#### DEPLOYMENTS.

15. A company may be deployed as skirmishers in two ways: forward, and by the flank.

16. The deployment forward will be adopted when the company is behind the line on which it is to be established as skirmishers: it will be deployed by the flank, when it finds itself already on that line.

17. Whenever a company is to be deployed as skirmishers, it will be divided into two platoons, and each platoon will be subdivided into two sections; the comrades in battle, forming groups of four men, will be careful to know and to sustain each other. The captain will assure himself that the files in the centre of each platoon and section are designated.

18. A company may be deployed as skirmishers on its right, left, or centre file, or on any other named file whatsoever. In this manner, skirmishers may be thrown forward with the greatest possible rapidity on any ground they may be required to occupy.

19. A chain of skirmishers ought generally to preserve their alignment, but no advantages which the ground may present should be sacrificed to attain this regularity.

20. The interval between skirmishers depends on the extent of ground to be covered; but in general, it is not proper that the groups of four men

should be removed more than forty paces from each other. The habitual distance between men of the same group in open grounds will be five paces; in no case will they lose sight of each other.

21. The front to be occupied to cover a battalion comprehends its front and the half of each interval which separates it from the battalion on its right and left. If a line, whose wings are not supported, should be covered by skirmishers, it will be necessary either to protect the flanks with skirmishers, or to extend them in front of the line so far beyond the wings as effectually to oppose any attempt which might be made by the enemy's skirmishers to disturb the flanks.

### To Deploy Forward

22. A company being at a halt or in march, when the captain shall wish to deploy it forward on the left file of the first platoon, holding the second platoon in reserve, he will command:

1. *First platoon—as skirmishers.*
2. *On the left file—take intervals.*
3. March (*or double quick*—March.)

23. At the first command, the second and third lieutenants will place themselves rapidly two paces behind the centres of the right and left sections of the first platoon; the fifth sergeant will move one pace in front of the centre of the first platoon, and will place himself between the two sections in the front rank as soon as the movement begins; the fourth sergeant will place himself on the left of the front rank of the same platoon, as soon as he can pass. The captain will indicate to this sergeant the point on which he wishes him to direct his march. The first lieutenant, placing himself before the centre of the second platoon, will command:

*Second platoon backward*—March.

24. At this command, the second platoon will step three paces to the rear, so as to unmask the flank of the first platoon. It will then be halted by its chief, and the second sergeant will place himself on the left, and the third sergeant on the right flank of this platoon.

25 At the command *march*, the left group of four men, conducted by the fourth sergeant, will direct itself on the point indicated; all the other groups of fours throwing forward briskly the left shoulder, will move diagonally to the front in double quick time, so as to gain to the right the space of twenty paces, which shall be the distance between each group and that immediately on its left. When the second group from the left shall arrive on a line with and twenty paces from the first, it will march straight to the front, conforming to the gait and direction of the first, keeping constantly on the same alignment and at twenty paces from it. The third group, and all the others will conform to what has just been prescribed for the second; they will arrive successively on the line. The right guide will arrive with the last group.

26. The left guide having reached the point where the left of the line should rest, the captain will command the skirmishers to halt; the men composing each group of fours will then immediately deploy at five paces from each other, and to the right and left of the front rank man or the even file in each group, the rear rank men placing themselves on the left of their file leaders. If any groups be not in line at the command *halt*, they will move up rapidly, conforming to what has just been described.

27. If, during the deployment, the line should be fired upon by the enemy, the captain may cause the groups of fours to deploy, as they gain their proper distances.

28. The line being formed, the non-commissioned officers on the right, left and centre of the platoon will place themselves ten paces in rear of the line,

and opposite the positions they respectively occupied. The chiefs of sections will promptly rectify any irregularities, and then place themselves twenty-five or thirty paces in rear of the centre of their sections. each having with him four men taken from the reserve. and also a bugler, who will repeat if necessary, the signals sounded by the captain.

29. Skirmishers should be particularly instructed to take advantage of any cover which the ground may offer, and should lie flat on the ground whenever such a movement is necessary to protect them from the fire of the enemy.   Regularity in the alignment should yield to this important advantage.

30. When the movement begins, the first lieutenant will face the second platoon *about*, and march it promptly, and by the shortest line, to about one hundred and fifty paces in rear of the centre of the line.  He will hold always at this distance, unless ordered to the contrary.

31. The reserve will conform itself to all the movements of the line. *This rule is general.*

32. Light troops will carry their bayonets habitually in the scabbard, and this rule applies equally to the skirmishers and the reserve ; whenever bayonets are required to be fixed. a particular signal will be given.  The captain will give a general superintendence to the whole deployment, and then promptly place himself about eighty paces in rear of the centre of the line.  He will have with him a bugler and four men taken from the reserve.

33. The deployment may be made on the right or the centre of the platoon, by the same commands, substituting the indication *right* or *centre*, for that of *left* file.

34. The deployment on the right or the centre will be made according to the principles prescribed above ; in this latter case. the centre of the platoon will be marked by the right group of fours in the second section ; the fifth sergeant will place himself on the right of this group, and serve as the guide of the platoon during the deployment.

35. In whatever manner the deployment be made, on the right, left, or centre, the men in each group of fours will always deploy at five paces from each other. and upon the front rank man of the even numbered file.  The deployments will habitually be made at twenty paces interval ; but if a greater interval be required, it will be indicated in the command.

36. If a company be thrown out as skirmishers, so near the main body as to render a reserve unnecessary. the entire company will be extended in the same manner. and according to the same principles, as for the deployment of a platoon   In this case the third lieutenant will command the fourth section. and a non-commissioned officer designated for that purpose, the seccond section; the fifth sergeant will act as centre guide ; the file closers will place themselves ten paces in rear of the line. and opposite their places in a line of battle. The first and second lieutenant will each have a bugler near him.

TO DEPLOY BY THE FLANK.

37. The company being at a halt. when the captain shall wish to deploy it by the flank, holding the first platoon in reserve, he will command :

1. *Second platoon—as skirmishers.*   2. *By the right flank—take intervals.*   3. MARCH
(or *double quick* MARCH.)

38. At the first command, the first and third lieutenants will place themselves respectively. two paces behind the centres of the first and second sections of the second platoon ; the fifth sergeant will place himself one pace in front of the centre of the second platoon ; the third sergeant. as soon as he can pass, will place himself on the right of the front rank of the same platoon.  The captain will indicate to him the point on which he wishes him to direct his march.  The chief of the first platoon will execute what has

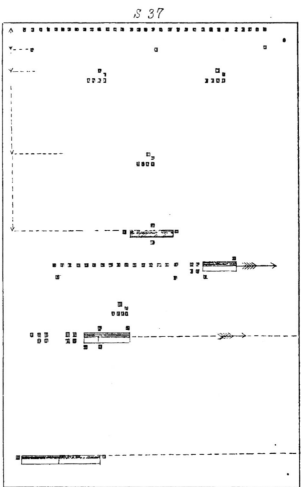

been prescribed for the chief of the second platoon. Nos. 23 and 24. The fourth sergeant will place himself on the left flank of the reserve, the first sergeant will remain on the right flank.

39. At the second command, the first and third lieutenants will place themselves two paces behind the left group of their respective sections.

40. At the command *march*, the second platoon will face to the right, and commence the movement; the left group of fours will stand fast, but will deploy as soon as there is room on its right, conforming to what has been prescribed No. 26; the third sergeant will place himself on the left of the right group to conduct it; the second group will halt at twenty paces from the one on its left, the third group at twenty paces from the second, and so on to the right. As the groups halt, they will face to the enemy, and deploy as has been explained for the left group.

41. The chiefs of sections will pay particular attention to the successive deployments of the groups, keeping near the group about to halt, so as to rectify any errors which may be committed. When the deployment is completed, they will place themselves thirty paces in rear of the centre of their sections, as has been heretofore prescribed. The non-commissioned officers will also place themselves as previously indicated.

42. As soon as the movement commences, the chief of the first platoon, causing it to face about, will move it as indicated No. 30.

43. The deployment may be made by the left flank according to the same principles, substituting *left flank* for *right flank*.

44. If the captain should wish to deploy the company upon the centre of one of the platoons, he will command:

1. *Second platoon—as skirmishers.* 2. *By the right and left flanks—take intervals.* 3. MARCH (*or double quick—*MARCH.)

45. At the first command, the officers and non-commissioned officers will conform to what has been prescribed No. 38.

46. At the second command, the first lieutenant will place himself behind the left group of the right section of the second platoon, the third lieutenant behind the right group of the left section of the same platoon.

47. At the command *march*, the right section will face to the right, the left section will face to the left, the group on the right of this latter section will stand fast. The two sections will move off in opposite directions: the third sergeant will place himself on the left of the right file to conduct it, the second sergeant on the right of the left file. The two groups nearest that which stands fast, will each halt at twenty paces from this group, and each of the other groups will halt at twenty paces from the group which is in rear of it. Each group will deploy as heretofore prescribed No. 40.

48. The first and third lieutenants will direct the movement, holding themselves always abreast of the group which is about to halt.

49. The captain can cause the deployment to be made on any named group whatsoever; in this case, the fifth sergeant will place himself before the group indicated, and the deployment will be made according to the principles heretofore prescribed.

50. The entire company may be also deployed, according to the same principles.

### TO EXTEND INTERVALS.

51. This movement, which is employed to extend a line of skirmishers, will be executed according to the principles prescribed for deployments.

52. If it be supposed that the line of skirmishers is at a halt, and that the captain wishes to extend it to the left, he will command:

1. *By the left flank,* (*so many paces*) *extend intervals.* 2. MARCH (*or double quick* —MARCH.)

53. At the command MARCH, the group on the right will stand fast, all the

other groups will face to the left, and each group will extend its interval to the prescribed distance by the means indicated No. 40.

54. The men of the same group will continue to preserve between each other the distance of five paces, unless the nature of the ground should render it necessary that they should close nearer, in order to keep in sight of each other. The intervals refer to the spaces between the groups, and not to the distances between the men in each group. The intervals will be taken from the right or left man of the neighboring group.

55. If the line of skirmishers be marching to the front, and the captain should wish to extend it to the right, he will command :

1. *On the left group, (so many paces) extend intervals.* 2. MARCH (or *double quick* —MARCH.)

56. The left group, conducted by the guide, will continue to march on the point of direction ; the other groups throwing forward the left shoulder, and taking the double quick step, will open their intervals to the prescribed distance, by the means indicated No. 25, conforming also to what is prescribed No. 54.

57. Intervals may be extended on the centre of the line, according to the same principles.

58. If, in extending intervals, it be intended that one company or platoon should occupy a line which had been previously occupied by two, the men of the company or platoon which is to retire, will fall successively to the rear as they are relieved by the extension of the intervals.

### To Close Intervals.

59. This movement, like that of opening intervals, will be executed according to the principles prescribed for the deployments.

60. If the line of skirmishers be halted, and the captain should wish to close intervals to the left, he will command :

1. *By the left flank (so many paces) close intervals.* 2. MARCH (or *double quick* MARCH).

61. At the command MARCH, the left group will stand fast, the other groups will face to the left and close to the prescribed distance, each group facing to the enemy as it attains its proper distance.

62. If the line be marching to the front, the captain will command :

1. *On the left group (so many paces) close intervals.* MARCH (or *double quick*— MARCH.)

63. The left group, conducted by the guide, will continue to move on in the direction previously indicated ; the other groups, advancing the right shoulder, will close to the left, until the intervals are reduced to the prescribed distance.

64. Intervals may be closed on the right, or on the centre, according to the same principles.

65. When intervals are to be closed up, in order to reinforce a line of skirmishers, so as to cause two companies to cover the ground which had been previously occupied by one, the new company will deploy so as to finish its movement at twenty paces in rear of the line it is to occupy, and the men will successively move upon that line, as they shall be unmasked by the men of the old company. The reserves of the two companies will unite behind the centre of the line.

### To Relieve a Company Deployed as Skirmishers.

66. When a company of skirmishers is to be relieved, the captain will be

advised of the intention, which he will immediately communicate to his first and second lieutenants.

67. The new company will execute its deployment forward, so as to finish the movement at about twenty paces in rear of the line.

68. Arrived at this distance, the men of the new company, by command of their captain, will advance rapidly a few paces beyond the old line and halt ; the new line being established, the old company will assemble on its reserve, taking care not to get into groups of fours until they are beyond the fire of the enemy.

69. If the skirmishers to be relieved are marching in retreat, the company thrown out to relieve them will deploy by the flank, as prescribed No. 38 and following. The old skirmishers will continue to retire with order, and having passed the new line, they will form upon the reverse.

## ARTICLE SECOND.

### TO ADVANCE.

*To advance in line, and to retreat in line.*

70. When a platoon or a company deployed as skirmishers is marching by the front, the guide will be habitually in the centre. No particular indication to this effect need be given in the commands, but if, on the contrary, it be intended that the directing guide should be on the right, or left, the command *guide right*, or *guide left*, will be given immediately after that of forward.

71. The captain, wishing the line of skirmishers to advance, will command :

1. *Forward.* 2· MARCH [or *double quick*—MARCH.]

72. This command will be repeated with the greatest rapidity by the chiefs of sections, and in case of need, by the sergeants. This rule is general, whether the skirmishers march by the front or by the flank.

73. At the first command, three sergeants will move briskly on the line, the first on the right, the second on the left, and the third in the centre.

74. At the command MARCH. the line will move to the front, the guide charged with the direction will move on the point indicated to him, the skirmishers will hold themselves aligned on this guide, and preserve their intervals towards him.

75. The chiefs of sections will march immediately behind their sections. so as to direct their movement.

76. The captain will give a general superintendence to the movement.

77. When he shall wish to halt the skirmishers, he will command :

#### HALT.

78. At this command, briskly repeated, the line will halt. The chiefs of sections will promptly rectify any irregularity in the alignment and intervals, and after taking every possible ad~antage which the ground may offer for protecting the men, they, with the three sergeants in the line, will retire to their proper places in rear.

79. The captain, wishing to march the skirmishers in retreat, will command :

1. *In retreat.* 2. MARCH [or *double quick*—MARCH.]

80. At the first command, the three sergeants will move on the line as prescribed No. 73.

81. At the command MARCH, the skirmishers will face about individually, and march to the rear, conforming to the principles prescribed No. 74.

82. The officers and sergeants will use every exertion to preserve order.

83. To halt the skirmishers marching in retreat, the captain will command :

### Halt.

84. At this command. the skirmishers will halt, and immediately face to the front.

85. The chiefs of sections and the three guides will each conform himself to what is prescribed No. 78.

### To Change Direction.

86. If the commander of a line of skirmishers shall wish to cause it to change direction to the right, he will command :

1. *Right wheel.* 2. March (or *double quick--*March )

87. At the command March, the right guide will mark time in his place ; the left guide will move in a circle to the right. and that he may properly regulate his movements, will occasionally cast his eyes to the right. so as to observe the direction of the line, and the nature of the ground to be passed over. The centre guide will also march in a circle to the right, and in order to conform his movements to the general direction. will take care that his steps are only half the length of the steps of the guide on the left.

88. The skirmishers will regulate the length of their steps by their distance from the marching flank, being less as they approach the pivot, and greater as they are removed from it ; they will often look to the marching flank, so as to preserve the direction and their intervals.

89. When the commander of the line shall wish to resume the direct march. he will command :

1 *Forward* 2. March

90. At the command March, the line will cease to wheel. and the skirmishers will move direct to the front ; the centre guide will march on the point which will be indicated to him.

91. If the captain should wish to halt the line. in place of moving it to the front, he will command :

### Halt.

92. At this command, the line will halt.

93. A change of direction to the left will be made according to the same principles. and by inverse means.

94. A line of skirmishers marching in retreat, will change direction by the same means, and by the same commands, as a line marching in advance ; for example, it the captain should wish to refuse his left, now become the right. he will command : 1. *Left wheel.* 2. March. At the command Halt, the skirmishers will face the enemy.

95. But if, instead of halting the line, the captain should wish to continue to march it in retreat,he will,when he judges the line has wheeled sufficiently. command :

1. *In retreat.* 2. March.

### To March by the Flank.

96. The captain, wishing the skirmishers to march by the right flank. will command :

1. *By the right flank.* 2. March (or *double quick—*March.)

97. At the first command, the three sergeants will place themselves on the line.

98. At the command March, the skirmishers will face to the right, and move off ; the right guide will place himself by the side of the leading man on the right to conduct him, and will march on the point indicated ; each

skirmisher will take care to follow exactly in the direction of the one immediately preceding him. and to preserve his distance.

99. The skirmishers may be marched by the left flank,according to the same principles. and by the same commands, substituting *left* for *right;* the left guide will place himself by the side of the leading man to conduct him,

100. If the skirmishers be marching by the flank. and the captain should wish to halt them, he will command :

HALT.

101. At this command, the skirmishers will halt and face to the enemy The officers and sergeants will conform to what has been prescribed No. 78.

102. The reserve should execute all the movements of the line, and be held always about one hundred and fifty paces from it. so as to be in position to second its operations.

103. When the chief of the reserve shall wish to march it in advance, he will command : 1. *Platoon forward.* 2. *Guide left.* 3. MARCH. If he should wish to march it in retreat, he will command : 1. *In retreat.* 2. MARCH. 3. *Guide right.* At the command HALT, it will reface to the enemy.

104. The men should be made to understand that the signals or commands, such as *forward,* mean that the skirmishers shall march on the enemy ; *in retreat,* that they shall retire, and to *the right or left flank,* that the men must face to the right or left, whatever may be their position.

105. If the skirmishers be marching by the flank, and the captain should wish to change direction to the right (or left), he will command : 1. *By file right* (or *left)*. 2. MARCH.

ARTICLE THIRD.

THE FIRINGS.

106. Skirmishers will either fire at a halt or marching.

To FIRE AT A HALT.

107. To cause this fire to be executed, the captain will command :

*Commence* —FIRING.

108. At this command, briskly repeated. the men of the front rank will commence firing ; they will reload rapidly. and hold themselves in readiness to fire again. During this time the men of the rear rank will come to a ready, and as soon as their respective file leaders have loaded, they will also fire and reload. The men of each file will thus continue the firing, conforming to this principle, that the one or the other shall always have his piece loaded.

109. Light troops should be always calm, so as to aim with accuracy ; they should, moreover, endeavor to estimate correctly the distance between themselves and the enemy to be hit, and thus be enabled to deliver their fire with the greater certainty of success.

110. Skirmishers will not remain in the same place whilst reloading. unless protected by accidents in the ground.

*To fire marching.*

111. This fire will be executed by the same commands as the fire at a halt.

112. At the command *commence firing,* if the line be advancing, the front rank man of every file will halt, fire. and reload before throwing himself forward. The rear rank man of the same file will continue to march, and after passing ten or twelve paces beyond his front rank man, will halt, come to a ready, select his object. and fire when his front rank man has loaded ; the fire will thus continue to be executed by each file ; the skirmishers will keep united, and endeavor, as much as possible, to preserve the general direction of the alignment.

14

113. If the line be marching in retreat, at the command *commence firing*, the front rank man of every file will halt, face to the enemy, fire, and then reload whilst moving to the rear ; the rear rank man of the same file will continue to march, and halt ten or twelve paces beyond his front rank man, face about, come to a ready, and fire, when his front rank man has passed him in retreat and loaded ; after which he will remove to the rear and reload ; the front rank man in his turn, after marching briskly to the rear, will halt at ten or twelve paces from the rear rank, face to the enemy, load his piece and fire, conforming to what has just been prescribed ; the firing will thus be continued.

114. If the company be marching by the right flank, at the command *commence firing*, the front rank man of every file will face to the enemy, step one pace forward, halt, and fire ; the rear rank man will continue to move forward. As soon as the front rank man has fired, he will place himself briskly behind his rear rank man and reload whilst marching. When he has loaded, the rear rank man will, in his turn, step one pace forward, halt, and fire, and returning to the ranks, will place himself behind his front rank man ; the latter, in his turn, will act in the same manner, observing the same principles. At the command, *cease firing*, the men of the rear rank will retake their original positions, if not already there.

115. If the company be marching by the left flank, the fire will be executed according to the same principles, but in this case, it will be the rear rank men who will fire first.

116. The following rules will be observed in the cases to which they apply.

117. If the line be firing at a halt, or whilst marching by the flank, at the command, *Forward—March*, it will be the men whose pieces are loaded, without regard to the particular rank to which they belong, who will move to the front. Those men whose pieces have been discharged, will remain in their places to load them before moving forward, and the firing will be continued agreeably to the principles prescribed No. 112.

118. If the line be firing either at a halt, advancing, or whilst marching by the flank, at the command, *In retreat—March*, the men whose pieces are loaded will remain faced to the enemy, and will fire in this position ; the men whose pieces are discharged will retreat loading them, and the fire will be continued agreeably to the principles prescribed No. 113.

119. If the line of skirmishers be firing either at a halt, advancing, or in retreat, at the command, *By the right (or left) flank—March*, the men whose pieces are loaded will step one pace out of the general alignment, face to the enemy, and fire in this position ; the men whose pieces are unloaded will face to the right (or left) and march in the direction indicated. The men who stepped out of the ranks will place themselves, immediately after firing, upon the general direction, and in rear of their front or rear rank men, as the case may be. The fire will be continued according to the principles prescribed No. 114.

120. Skirmishers will be habituated to load their pieces whilst marching ; but they will be enjoined to halt always an instant, when in the act of charging cartridge, and priming.

121. They should be practised to fire and load kneeling, lying down, and sitting, and much liberty should be allowed in these exercises, in order that they should be executed in the manner found to be most convenient. Skirmishers should be cautioned not to forget that, in whatever position they may load, it is important that the piece should be placed upright before ramming, in order that the entire charge of powder may reach the bottom of the bore.

122. In commencing the fire, the men of the same rank should not all fire at once, and the men of the same file should be particular that one or the other of them be always loaded.

123. In retreating, the officer commanding the skirmishers should seize on every advantage which the ground may present, for arresting the enemy as long as possible.

124. At the signal to *cease firing*, the captain will see that the order is

promptly obeyed ; but the men who may not be loaded, will load. If the line be marching, it will continue the movement ; but the man of each file who happens to be in front, will wait until the man in rear shall be abreast with him.

125. It a line of skirmishers be firing advancing, at the command. *halt*, the line will re-form upon the skirmishers who are in front ; when the line is retreating, upon the skirmishers who are in rear.

126. Officers should watch with the greatest possible vigilance over a line of skirmishers ; in battle, they should neither carry a rifle or fowling piece. In all the firings, they, as well as the sergeants, should see that order and silence are preserved, and that the skirmishers do not wander imprudently : they should especially caution them to be calm and collected ; not to fire until they distinctly perceived the objects at which they aim, and are sure that those objects are within proper range. Skirmishers should take advantage promptly, and with intelligence, of all shelter, and of all accidents of the ground, to conceal themselves from the view of the enemy, and to protect themselves from his fire. It may often happen, that intervals are momentarily lost when several men near each other find a common shelter ; but when they quit this position they should immediately resume their intervals and their places in line, so that they may not, by crowding, needlessly expose themselves to the fire of the enemy.

ARTICLE FOURTH.

THE RALLY.— *To Form Column.*

127. A company deployed as skirmishers, is rallied in order to oppose the enemy with better success : the rallies are made at a run, and with bayonets fixed ; when ordered to rally, the skirmishers fix bayonets without command.

128. There are several ways of rallying, which the chief of the line will adopt according to circumstances.

129. If the line, marching or at a halt, be merely disturbed by scattered horsemen, it will not be necessary to fall back on the reserve, but the captain will cause bayonets to be fixed. If the horsemen should, however, advance to charge the skirmishers, the captain will command, *rally by fours.* The line will halt, if marching, and the four men of each group will execute this rally in the following manner ; the front rank men of the even numbered file will take the position of *guard against cavalry* ; the rear rank man of the odd numbered file will also take the position of *guard against cavalry*, turning his back to him, his right foot thirteen inches from the right foot of the former and parallel to it ; the front rank man of the odd file, and the rear rank man of the even file, will also place themselves back to back, taking a like position, and between the two men already established, facing to the right and left ; the right feet of the four men will be brought together, forming a square, and serving for mutual support. The four men in each group will come to a ready, fire as occasion may offer, and load without moving their feet

130. The captain and chiefs of sections will each cause the four men who constitute his guard to form square, the men separating so as to enable him and the bugler to place themselves in the centre. The three sergeants will each promptly place himself in the group nearest him in the line of skirmishers.

131. Whenever the captain shall judge these squares too weak, but should wish to hold his position by strengthening his line, he will command :

*Rally by Sections.*

132. At this command, the chiefs of sections will move rapidly on the centre group of their respective sections, or on any other interior group whose position might offer a shelter, or other particular advantage ; the skirmishers will

collect rapidly at a run on this group, and without distinction of numbers. The men composing the group on which the formation is made, will immediately form square, as heretofore explained, and elevate their pieces, the bayonets uppermost, in order to indicate the point on which the rally is to be made. The other skirmishers as they arrive, will occupy and fill the open angular spaces between these four men, and successively rally around this first nucleus, and in such a manner as to form rapidly a compact circle. The skirmishers will take as they arrive, the position of charge bayonet, the point of the bayonet more elevated, and will cock their pieces in this position. The movement concluded, the two exterior ranks will fire as occasion may offer, and load without moving their feet.

133. The captain will move rapidly with his guard, wherever he may judge his presence is most necessary.

134. The officers and sergeants will be particular to observe that the rally is made in silence, and with promptitude and order ; that some pieces in each of their subdivisions be at all times loaded. and that the fire is directed on those points only where it will be the most effective.

135. If the reserve should be threatened, it will form in a circle around its chief.

136. If the captain, or commander of a line of skirmishers formed of many platoons, should judge that the rally by section does not offer sufficient resistance, he will cause the rally by platoons to be executed. and for this purpose, will command :

*Rally by platoons.*

137. This movement will be executed according to the same principles, and by the same means, as the rally by sections. The chiefs of platoon will conform to what has been prescribed for the chiefs of section.

138. The captain wishing to rally the skirmishers on the reserve, will command :

*Rally on the reserve.*

139. At this command, the captain will move briskly on the reserve ; the officer who commands it will take immediate steps to form square ; for this purpose, he will cause the half sections on the flanks to be thrown perpendicularly to the rear ; he will order the men to come to a ready.

140. The skirmishers of each section. taking the run, will form rapidly into groups, and upon that man of each group who is nearest the centre of the section. These groups will direct themselves diagonally towards each other, and in such manner as to form into sections with the greatest rapidity while moving to the rear ; the officers and sergeants will see that this formation is made in proper order. and the chiefs will direct their sections upon the reserve, taking care to unmask it to the right and left. As the skirmishers arrive, they will continue and complete the formation of the square begun by the reserve, closing in rapidly upon the latter, without regard to their places in line ; they will come to a ready without command, and fire upon the enemy ; which will also be done by the reserve as soon as it is unmasked by the skirmishers.

141. If a section should be closely pressed by cavalry while retreating, its chief will command HALT ; at this command, the men will form rapidly into a compact circle around the officer, who will re-form his section, and resume the march, the moment he can do so with safety.

142. The formation of the square in a prompt and efficient manner requires coolness and activity on the part of both officers and sergeants.

143. The captain will also profit by every moment of respite which the enemy's cavalry may leave him ; as soon as he can, he will endeavor to place himself beyond the reach of their charges, either by gaining a position where he may defend himself with advantage, or by returning to the corps to which

he belongs. For this purpose, being in square, he will cause the company to break into column by platoons at half distance : to this effect, he will command :

1. *Form column.* 2. MARCH.

144. At the command MARCH, each platoon will dress on its centre, and the platoon which was facing to the rear will face about without command. The guides will place themselves on the right and left of their respective platoons, those of the second platoon will place themselves at half distance from those of the first, counting from the rear rank. These dispositions being made, the captain can move the column in whatever direction he may judge proper.

145. If he wishes to march it in retreat, he will command:

1. *In retreat.* 2. MARCH (*or double quick*—MARCH).

146. At the command MARCH, the column will immediately face by the rear rank, and move off in the opposite direction. As soon as the column is in motion, the captain will command :

3. *Guide right* (*or left.*)

147. He will indicate the direction to the leading guide ; the guides will march at their proper distances, and the men will keep aligned.

148. It again threatened by cavalry, the captain will command :

1. *Form square.* 2. MARCH.

149. At the command MARCH, the column will halt ; the first platoon will face about briskly, and the outer half sections of each platoon will be thrown perpendicularly to the rear, so as to form the second and third fronts of the square. The officers and sergeants will promptly rectify any irregularities which may be committed.

150. If he should wish to march the column in advance, the captain will command :

1. *Form column.* 2. MARCH.

151. Which will be executed as prescribed No. 144.

152. The column being formed, the captain will command :

1. *Forward.* 2. MARCH (*or double quick*—MARCH). 3. *Guide left* (*or right.*)

153. At the second command, the column will move forward, and at the third command, the men will take the touch of elbows to the side of the guide.

154. It the captain should wish the column to gain ground to the right or left, he will do so by rapid wheels to the side opposite the guide, and for this purpose, will change the guide whenever it may be necessary.

155. If a company be in column by platoon, at half distance, right in front, the captain can deploy the first platoon as skirmishers by the means already explained ; but if it should be his wish to deploy the second platoon forward on the centre file, leaving the first platoon in reserve, he will command :

1. *Second platoon—as skirmishers.* 2. *On the centre file—take intervals.* 3. MARCH (*or double quick*—MARCH.)

156. At the first command, the chief of the first platoon will caution his platoon to stand fast ; the chiefs of sections of the second platoon will place themselves before the centre of their sections : the fifth sergeant will place himself one pace in front of the centre of the second platoon.

157. At the second command, the chief of the right section, second platoon, will command : *Section, right face ;* the chief of the left section : *Section, left face.*

158. At the command MARCH, these sections will move off briskly in opposite directions, and having unmasked the first platoon, the chiefs of sections will respectively command : *By the left flank*—MARCH. and *By the right flank—*

MARCH; and as soon as these sections arrive on the aligment of the first platoon, they will command : *As skirmishers—MARCH.* The groups will then deploy according to prescribed principles, on the right group of the left section, which will be directed by the fifth sergeant on the point indicated.

159. If the captain should wish the deployment made by the flank, the second platoon will be moved to the front by the means above stated, and halted after passing some steps beyond the alignment of the first platoon ; the deployment will then be made by the flank according to the principles prescribed.

160. When one or more platoons are deployed as skirmishers, and the captain should wish to rally them on the battalion, he will command :

Rally on the battalion.

161. At this command, the skirmishers and the reserve, no matter what position the company to which they belong may occupy in order of battle, will rapidly unmask the front of the battalion, directing themselves in a run towards its nearest flank, and then form in its rear.

162. As soon as the skirmishers have passed beyond the line of file closers, the men will take the quick step, and the chief of each platoon or section will re-form his subdivision, and place it in column behind the wing on which it is rallied ; and at ten paces from the rank of file closers. These subdivisions will not be moved except by order of the commander of the battalion, who may, if he thinks proper, throw them into line of battle at the extremities of the line, or in the intervals between the battalions

163. If many platoons should be united behind the same wing of a battalion, or behind any shelter whatsoever, they should be formed always in close column, or into column at half distance.

164. When the battalion, covered by a company of skirmishers, shall be formed into square, the platoons and sections of the covering company will be directed by their chiefs to the rear of the square, which will be opened at the angles to receive the skirmishers, who will be then formed into close column by platoons in rear of the first front of the square.

165. If circumstances should prevent the angles of the square from being opened, the skirmishers will throw themselves at the feet of the front rank men, the right knee on the ground, the butt of the piece resting on the thigh, the bayonet in a threatening position. A part may also place themselves about the angles, where they can render good service by defending the sectors without fire.

166. If the battalion on which the skirmishers are rallied, be in column ready to form square, the skirmishers will be formed into close column by platoon, in rear of the centre of the third division, and at the command, *Form square—MARCH,* they will move forward and close on the buglers.

167. When skirmishers have been rallied by platoon or section behind the wings of a battalion, and it be wished to deploy them again to the front, they will be marched by the flank towards the intervals on the wings, and be then deployed so as to cover the front of the battalion

168. When platoons or sections, placed in the interior of squares or columns, are to be deployed, they will be marched out by the flanks, and then thrown forward, as is precribed No. 157 ; as soon as they shall have unmasked the column or square, they will be deployed, the one on the right, the other on the left file.

The assembly.

169. A company deployed as skirmishers will be assembled when there is no longer danger of its being disturbed; the assembly will be made habitually in quick time.

170. The captain wishing to assemble the skirmishers on the reserve will command :

S. 178.

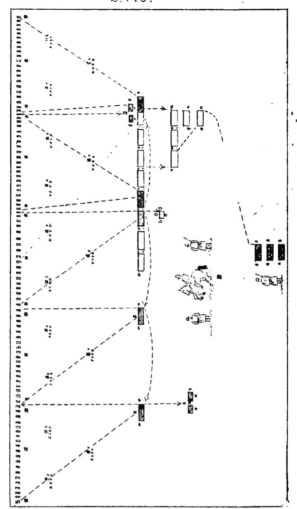

*Assemble on the reserve.*

171. At this command, the skirmishers will assemble by groups of fours; the front rank men will place themselves behind their rear rank men ; and each group of fours will erect itself on the reserve, where each will take its proper place in the ranks. When the company is re-formed, it will re-join the battalion to which it belongs.

172. It may be also proper to assemble the skirmishers on the centre, or on the right or left of the line, either marching, or at a halt.

173. If the captain should wish to assemble them on the centre while marching, he will command :

*Assemble on the centre.*

174. At this command, the centre guide will continue to march directly to the front on the point indicated ; the front rank man of the directing file will follow the guide, and be covered by his rear rank man ; the other two comrades of this group, and likewise those on their left, will march diagon-, ally, advancing the left shoulder and accelerating the gait so as to re-form the groups while drawing nearer and nearer the directing file ; the men of the right section will unite in the same manner into groups, and then upon the directing file, throwing forward the right shoulder. As they successively unite on the centre, the men will bring their pieces to the right shoulder.

175. To assemble on the right or left file will be executed according to the same principles.

176. The assembly of a line marching in retreat will also be executed according to the same principles. the front rank men marching behind their rear rank men.

177. To assemble the line of skirmishers at a halt, and on the line they occupy, the captain will give the same command ; the skirmishers will face to the right or left, according as they should march by the right or left flank, re-form the groups while marching and thus arrive on the file which served as the point of formation. As they successively arrive, the skirmishers will support arms.

## ARTICLE *FIFTH.*

TO DEPLOY A BATTALION AS SKIRMISHERS, AND TO RALLY THIS BATTALION.

*To deploy the battalion as skirmishers.*

178. A battalion being in line of battle, if the commander should wish to deploy it on the right of the sixth company, holding the three right companies in reserve, he will signify his intention to the lieutenant colonel and adjutant, and also to the major, who will be directed to take charge of the reserve. He will point out to the lieutenant colonel the direction he wishes to give the line, as well as the point where he wishes the right of the sixth company to rest, and to the commander of the reserve the place he may wish it established.

179. The lieutenant colonel will move· rapidly in front of the right of the sixth company, and the adjutant in front of the left of the same company. The commander of the reserve will dispose of it in the manner to be herein-after indicated.

180. The colonel will command :

1. *First* (or *second*) *platoon—as skirmishers.*

2. *On the right of the sixth company —take intervals.*

3. MARCH (or *double quick*—MARCH.)

181. At the scond command, the captains of the fifth and sixth companies will prepare to deploy the first platoons of their respective companies, the sixth on its right, the fifth on its left file.

182. The captain of the fourth company will face it to the right, the aud captains of the seventh and eighth companies will face their respective companies to the left.

183. At the command *march*, the movement will commence. The platoons of the fifth and sixth companies will deploy forward; the right guide of the sixth will march on the point which will be indicated to him by the lieutenant colonel.

184. The company which has faced to the right, and also the companies which have faced to the left, will march straight forward. The fourth company will take an interval of one hundred paces counting from the left of the fifth, and its chiefs will deploy its first platoon on its left file. The seventh and eighth companies will each take an interval of one hundred paces. counting from the first file of the company, which is immediately on its right; and the chiefs of these companies will afterward deploy their first platoons on the right file.

185. The guides who conduct the files on which the deployment is made, should be careful to direct themselves towards the outer man of the neighboring company, already deployed as skirmishers; or if the company has not finished its deployment, they will judge carefully the distance which may still be required to place all these files in line, and will then march on the point thus marked out. The companies, as they arrive on the line, will align themselves on those already deployed.

186. The lieutenant-colonel and adjutant will follow the deployment, the one on the right, the other on the left; the movement concluded. they will place themselves near the colonel.

187. The reserves of the companies will be established in echellon, in the following manner; the reserve of the sixth company will be placed one hundred and fifty paces in rear of the right of this company; the reserves of the fourth and fifth companies, united, opposite the centre of their line of skirmishers, and thirty paces in advance of the reserve of the sixth company: the reserves of the seventh and eighth companies, also united, opposite the centre of their line of skirmishers, and thirty paces farther to the rear than the reserve of the sixth company.

188. The major commanding the companies composing the reserve, on receiving an order from the colonel to that effect. will march these companies thirty paces to the rear, and will then ploy them into column by company, at half distance; after which, he will conduct the column to the point which shall have been indicated to him.

189. The colonel will have a general superintendence of the movement; and when it is finished, will move to a point in rear of the line whence his view may best embrace the parts, in order to direct their movements.

190. If, instead of deploying forward, it be desired to deploy by the flank. the sixth and fifth companies will be moved to the front ten or twelve paces, halted, and deployed by the flank, the one on the right, the other on the left file, by the means already indicated. Each of the other companies will be marched by the flank; and as soon as the last file of the company, next towards the direction, shall have taken its interval, it will be moved upon the line established by the fifth and sixth companies, halted, and deployed.

191. In the preceding example, it has been supposed that the battalion was in order of battle; but if in column, it would be deployed as skirmishers by the same commands and according to the same principles.

192. If the deployment is to be made *forward*, the directing company, as soon as it is unmasked, will be moved ten or twelve paces in front of the head of the column, and will be then deployed on the file indicated. Each of the other companies will take its interval to the right or left, and deploy as soon as it is taken.

193. If the deployment is to be made by the flank, the directing company will be moved in the same manner to the front, as soon as it is unmasked. and

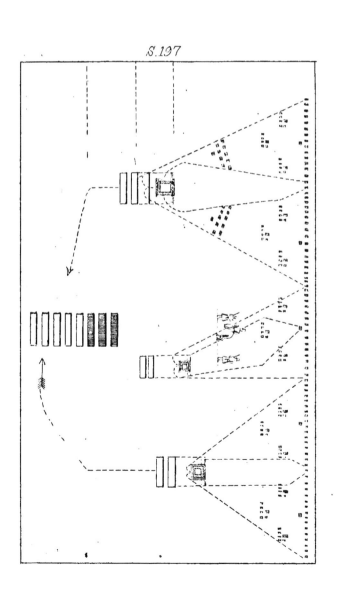

will then be halted and deployed by the flank, on the file indicated. Each of the other companies will be marched by the flank, and when its interval is taken, will be moved on the line, halted, and deployed as soon as the company next towards the direction shall have finished its deployment.

194. It has been prescribed to place the reserves in echellon, in order that they may, in the event of a rally, be able to protect themselves without injuring each other ; and the reserves of two contiguous companies have been united, in order to diminish the number of the echellons, and to increase their capacity for resisting cavalry.

195. The echellons, in the example given, descend from right to left, but they may, on an indication from the colonel to that effect, be posted on the same principle, so as to descend from left to right.

196. When the color company is to be deployed as skirmishers, the color, without its guard, will be detached, and remain with the battalion reserve.

*The rally.*

197. The colonel may cause all the various movements prescribed for a company, to be executed by the battalion, and by the same commands and the same signals. When he wishes to rally the battalion, he will cause the *rally on the battalion* to be sounded, and will so dispose his reserve as to protect this movement.

198. The companies deployed as skirmishers will be rallied in squares on their respective reserves ; each reserve of two contiguous companies will form the first front of the square, throwing to the rear the sections on the flank ; the skirmishers who arrive first will complete the lateral fronts, and the last the fourth front. The officers and sergeants will superintend the rally. and as fast as the men arrive, they will form them into two ranks, without regard to height, and cause them to face outwards.

199. The rally being effected, the commanders of squares will profit by any interval of time the cavalry may allow for putting them in safety, either by marching upon the battalion reserves, or by seizing an advantageous position : to this end, each of the squares will be formed into column, and march in this order ; and if threatened anew, it will halt, and again form itself into square.

200. As the companies successively arrive near the battalion reserve each will re-form as promptly as possible, and without regard to designation or number, take place in the column next in rear of the companies already in it.

201. The battalion reserve will also form square, if itself threatened by cavalry, In this case, the companies in marching towards it, will place themselves promptly in the sectors without fire, and thus march on the squares.

[END OF INSTRUCTIONS FOR SKIRMISHERS.]

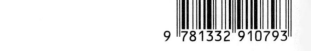
9 781332 910793

Printed by BoD™in Norderstedt, Germany